AUTOCIZE

AUTOCIZE

by JAY DAVID, *pseud.*

Bill Adler

WILLIAM MORROW AND COMPANY, INC.

NEW YORK   1979

Copyright © 1979 by Bill Adler Books, Inc.

Library of Congress Cataloging in Publication Data

———
    Autocize.

    1. Exercise.   2. Sitting position.   3. Automobile driving—Physiological aspects.   I. Title.
RA781.A3   613.7'1   78-23751
ISBN 0-688-03399-7

BOOK DESIGN   CARL WEISS

Printed in the United States of America.

First Edition

1   2   3   4   5   6   7   8   9   10

CONTENTS

2081880

6 /

PART III

PART

I

FINDING
FLAB

"Necessity is the mother of invention" is not an original statement, but it is an apt one in my case. Autocize came about because of a need—a need to exercise. However much I needed exercise, I did not have the time; the only free time available to me was the hours I spent in my car. But I am getting ahead of myself. Just as it took me a while to realize the possibilities my car offered, it took me a while to notice my poor physical condition.

For a long time I considered myself lucky—I did not have a weight problem. My weight never varied by more than 3 pounds from my norm of 170 pounds. In the last fifteen years I never weighed more than 173 or less than 167 pounds. This fact gave me a false sense of security as far as my physical condition was concerned because everyone I knew—friends, relatives, business associates, even my wife—was concerned about his or her weight. For a while it seemed as though everyone I spoke to weighed too much and was following a diet.

But there is more to good physical condition than the proper weight. There is also good muscle tone, and this was something I ignored. If my four-year-old daughter, Lauren, had not announced one evening, "You know why I like sitting on your lap, Daddy? Because your stomach's so soft and squishy. It's better than a pillow," I might still be unaware of my poor muscle tone. Once my flabby stomach had been pointed out, I took a good, long look at me. Sure enough, those firm, hard muscles which I had been so proud of during my college days were no more.

Not only did I have what is commonly, but not elegantly, called a beer gut, but I also had fleshy arms and sagging jowls. And I was only thirty-five years old! There is, as far as I know, only one way to firm up flabby muscles, and that way is exercise.

At this point I began to envy people who had weight problems. All they had to do was follow a diet. You don't have to find time for that; you just adhere to a particular way of eating. Exercise is something else; it requires time. And I don't have a lot of time at my disposal. More precisely, I don't have time to spend exercising, and this is due to my current life-style.

I sell highly sophisticated computers. Sounds easy, I know, but it takes a lot of time. For one thing, my clients are widely scattered, so I spend a lot of time in my car. It's not unusual for me to leave my house at six-thirty in the morning so that I can make a nine-thirty meeting with a customer in a distant city. And because the equipment I sell and service is not exactly cheap, making the sale might be an all-day session with half a dozen company officials. By five o'clock I might find myself three hours from home.

Once I do get home, I'm tired. I want to relax, talk to my wife and kids, read the paper, and watch a little television. Even those evenings when I do get home at a decent hour, I still want time for my family. My eight-year-old son is very much into building models, and I try to help whenever I can. That takes time, but that hour or so is too valuable and too important to drop from my daily schedule.

Of course, there are weekends and holidays, but again that time is spoken for. Because the equipment I sell is highly technical and always changing, there is a lot of reading to do. There are reports to write. What model is selling or not selling and why. What the customer likes or dislikes about the equipment. What improvements could be made in future models.

I do, however, play a lot of golf and usually with a customer. Yet those golf games are not as physically worthwhile as they might be because I use a golf cart. Briefly I toyed with the idea of substituting a more vigorous sport for golf, a sport like tennis. That, on second thought, proved impractical. A lot of business is discussed while we tool around in that golf cart. Try talking up a product while you're flying around a tennis court. Golf it had to be when business was on the agenda, but that left me with the golf cart hurdle. A few of the men I knew genuinely believed that the cart was necessary for their health and well-being, especially those with histories of heart trouble. They were ever so careful about their health, except when it was their turn to swing a club. Most of the men I play golf with, however, use a cart because they don't want to walk. I was not going to risk antagonizing a good customer by insisting that we walk the course. After all, I have a family to support and bills to pay.

By the time I outlined my schedule and studied it there didn't seem to be any place where I could fit in some daily exercise. That fact frustrated me, but at least I could console myself with the thought that I was not alone. Most of my friends and relatives freely admitted that they needed physical exercise; they also insisted that they had no time for a regular program of physical activity. As a close friend and neighbor of mine explained, "Sure I need exercise. Who doesn't? But when? That's the problem. The only time I have that is my own is when I'm driving back and forth to the train station. That twenty minutes each way is it. If I could exercise during that time, I would."

A cousin of mine expressed much the same sentiments when she said, "With three small children who require constant chauffeuring, I'm lucky that I have time to take a shower, much less exercise. If I'm not carting my son to Little League practice, I'm driving my daughter to dancing class or taking the baby to the doctor's. Between the kids and the errands, I might as well live in my station wagon, but who exercises in a station wagon?"

The son of one of my friends added his voice. Jerry had decided to become a long-distance truck driver, work he loved, but the job had its disadvantages. "I probably need exercise more than most people," he told me, "but I've got a delivery schedule to meet. At the end of a run I just want to sleep, not exercise. What makes it really bad is the fact that during a trip I eat at these fast food places. Pizzas, hamburgers, french fries—a lot of empty calories. It's beginning to show. My weight is going up, but when do I have time to exercise? * If I weren't driving, I'd probably have the time."

The list of people who needed, who wanted exercise, but who had no time, could go on and on. And like me, they all seemed to spend a lot of time behind the wheel of a car, truck, or van.

"There has to be an hour somewhere," I kept telling myself. "If not a whole hour, then at least thirty minutes." Yet no matter how hard I looked, I couldn't find those needed minutes. I couldn't find the time because I was looking for consecutive minutes. It never occurred to me to think in terms of a minute here and a minute there. That was a big mistake. Several weeks went by before I realized the mistake I, and so many other people, had made.

I was on my way home one evening when I ran into a massive traffic jam. Some sort of repair work was being done on the expressway I use, and three lanes of rush-hour traffic had to merge into one lane. To make matters worse, the re-

---

* See Chapter 15 for a discussion of "eating on the run."

pair work was being done just before an entrance ramp. As the three lanes of traffic were merging into one lane, cars were also trying to merge into traffic. It was a nightmare! I'd creep forward a few feet and then sit in the car for three or four minutes going nowhere and doing nothing.

"No wonder nobody has time to exercise," I fumed to myself. "Look at all the time that is wasted while in a car. Just sitting. Doing nothing of any value." That's when it hit me. All the time that people spend in a car "doing nothing." A nice chunk of time.

"Of course, a good deal of that time is spent in driving," I reminded myself. "I have to pay attention to what I'm doing. But how much time do I, and other people, spend in traffic jams, at red lights, in parking spaces waiting for someone?" I decided it had to be at least thirty minutes a day, if not more. Time, I had to admit, that had been wasted by me and a lot of other people as well. Only that morning, I had been waiting in my car for a colleague of mine who had dashed into a candy store to buy a pack of cigarettes. I had spent those two or three minutes adding up license plate numbers in my head. Why couldn't I have put that time to better use by doing a few exercises? There was nothing to stop me.

At last I found the solution to the problem of no time for exercises. Instead of just wasting time while sitting in a car, I could put that time to good use. Once I had the idea, I checked it out with a close friend of mine, a college roommate who became a physical education teacher. After the two of us researched the subject, we discovered it was possible to exercise in a car. There is a large variety of stretching, isometric, and yoga motions that can be done easily—and safely—in an automobile. For want of a better description, I started to refer to my physical fitness program as autocizing.

We all view an automobile as a vehicle of transportation, but as a vehicle to tone up loose, flabby muscles! It most certainly is! Not only does an automobile provide the time for a shape-up program, but it also provides the space—more than most people realize.

So if you are in the same position I was in awhile back— you know you need some regular exercise, but you can't seem to find the time—autocizing could be the answer. Indeed, it probably is, because autocize is for everybody.

CHAPTER

2

THERE'S A
LOT TO LIKE

Autocizing is a head-to-toe physical tune-up that has a number of advantages when compared to the more traditional forms of exercising. The most obvious advantage, of course, is time. There is no longer the need to squeeze out thirty or sixty minutes from an already-crowded schedule so you can exercise. Anyone who drives a car (or rides in one, but more about this later) has time to autocize. And for those of you who still have doubts, do what I did. Keep a record, for a week, of the time you spend in a car when you are not *actually* driving. While I used a stopwatch, you can use an ordinary watch with a sweep-second hand. But there is more to autocize than the time factor.

A lot of exercise programs require special equipment: things like mats, barbells, jump ropes, and even special clothes. The need for this equipment often keeps people from an exercise program. And who can blame them? I can't, because I share their feelings. This stuff is expensive. Today most of us are looking for ways to cut back on spending, not to increase it. Too, this equipment takes up room. Nearly everyone needs more living space than he has. My family and I certainly do. We just don't have the space available for a home gym.

Autocizing makes no such demands. There is no special equipment to buy, and there are no storage problems to solve. The only thing you need to start autocizing is an automobile, or a truck, or a van. "Of course, Jay," a friend pointed out while I was explaining autocize, "there are spas and exercise clubs available for folks who don't want to buy or store equipment." That's true, but that nagging question of time creeps back in. People who can't find an hour or so to exercise in their own homes aren't going to find it any easier to get over to a gym or club. Too, there is the expense factor. These places all charge a fee, and not everyone is anxious to pay it.

It doesn't take much to put a stumbling block in the way of an exercise program, does it? Autocize isn't like that. You don't have to go anywhere special. You just have to be in a car. In short, nearly everyone can autocize without having to find time, spend money, or turn his life and living space upside down unless he chooses to do so.

These exercises can also be used in conjunction with other fitness programs. Autocize makes a perfect supplement for those who do work out at home or belong to a gym. So even if you already have a fitness program, consider autocize. It's a great way to make the best use of all your available time.

Even though we all realize the need for physical fitness, most of us avoid exercise whenever we can, partially because we as human beings have a streak of laziness within us. We are always looking for ways to save physical energy. As a salesman, I know this well. Label any product as a "step saver," and people really sit up and take notice. Point out the work-saving features, and people can't buy the product fast enough. But laziness is not the only reason so many people avoid exercise.

There is also the fact that we do not like to be bored. We are thinking creatures, and as such, we need to be kept interested. And frankly a lot of exercise is just plain boring. That's why so many start off on this fourteen-day shape-up program and that twenty-one-day fitness binge and lose interest after two days. The whole thing becomes dull and mind-deadening. All those good intentions and the initial enthusiasm fade away quickly. The cause? A loss of interest.

Who, after all, is really fascinated by the prospect of doing thirty push-ups every single day? Or jogging half a mile? Or pedaling away on an exercise bicycle? Especially when there is that feeling of "I have to do this!" That sense of obligation gets to many of us very quickly. It's a fast turnoff if there ever was one. "I want to do this" is the best way to inspire enthusiasm.

Autocizes are not boring. They all are accomplished in a matter of minutes. In some cases, in a matter of seconds. And rather than create boredom, they actually serve to relieve it. That, in turn, makes you a better driver. The driver who is not bored is more alert.

Autocizing can also help relieve tension. A driver is more relaxed if he autocizes. The alert, relaxed driver is a safer driver. And all this brings me to what is perhaps the greatest advantage of autocizing—safety. Let me illustrate this point with a little story.

It is 5:45 on a weekday evening in a major American city. The roads leading from the city to the various suburbs are jammed. Traffic is moving at a crawl. One particular artery seems to be moving even more slowly than the others. Most of the drivers don't know why; they can't see the disabled car blocking one lane and the owner trying, unsuccessfully, to push the vehicle off the highway onto the shoulder.

This is a common weekday scene on any American highway during the rush hour. Chances are you yourself often face this situation. How do you react to it? Would you tense up? A lot of people would. My accountant, Bob M., used to do just that.

"As soon as I hit a traffic jam with cars creeping along at half a mile an hour, I'd start boiling over at the lack of progress. I'd start taking chances that I shouldn't. Cutting somebody off to change lanes. Not that it did me much good;

the traffic would be just as slow. A couple of times I came close to having an accident because of what I was doing. By the time I got home I'd have a headache, maybe a stomachache, and definitely a lousy disposition. My wife and kids never looked forward to those first ten minutes when I got home."

Tensing up is one reaction to a traffic jam. Getting bored is another. Larry used to be that way. He's a fellow I play golf with. One Saturday morning he showed up with his fender half gone. "What happened to your car?" I asked.

"Last night on the way home," he explained, "there was a lot of traffic, and after the first twenty feet I got bored. I just stopped paying attention. I was sort of glancing through the paper, and every once in a while I'd take my foot off the brake and let the car creep forward a bit. It always worked before, but not last night. I let the car creep too much and locked fenders with a guy who was merging in. Never noticed him at all. It could have been worse, though. Frankly I was just too bored with the traffic situation to pay attention."

Being tensed up or bored is not the way to drive a car. It is just too dangerous, and these men agreed with me when we talked about it. The problem, though, was how to avoid tension and boredom while we drive cars. The solution was to autocize.

As Bob told me after he acquired the autocize habit, "Jay, doing a few exercises when traffic comes to a standstill keeps me sane on the way home. Rather than tense up, I begin to unwind. No more boiling over about the lack of progress, something I can't do anything about anyway. Now I get home relaxed, and my family is glad to see me."

Larry came to the same conclusion. "Rather than let my attention wander," he said, "I pay attention to traffic. So many of the autocizes can be done without diverting your attention from the task at hand—driving."

But there are further advantages. Autocizing is a fitness program for almost everybody. The amount of time you spend in a car is not important. The driver who spends just a few minutes each day in a car, like the commuter who goes from his house to the train station, can autocize as easily as the driver who spends several hours a day behind the wheel. People who make several short trips in the course of a day can also autocize. So the housewife who spends her time shuttling back and forth in her car can put herself into shape.

The type of vehicle you drive is not important. All makes and models—station wagons, sedans, convertibles (if you're lucky enough to own one), compacts, vans, and trucks—are great for autocizing. Of course, some autocizes are more suited to a station wagon than to a compact, but more about that later.

When I said everybody could take up autocizing, I meant it. Even people who do not drive can autocize. This program can be used by passengers as well as by drivers. And you do not necessarily have to be a passenger in a car, either, as one of my wife's friends discovered.

Just after she began autocizing, Maria called and happily announced, "It's a great help. What I find especially helpful about autocize is that you don't necessarily need a car. Oh, I realize that the whole idea is to do these exercises in an automobile, but I don't drive. I doubt that I ever will, but I do travel a lot. My job has me running from one part of the country to another, but whether I'm in a train or on a plane, I can do some autocizes."

Autocize is a fitness program that can complement your personality as well as your personal goals. I have to admit that the complementary features did not originate with me. A young college student first pointed them out to me. Hank, who has a part-time job driving a cab, raved about autocizes because they allowed him to have what he termed "super rap sessions" with his passengers. Naturally I asked how, and he explained, "A lot of my fares aren't too interested in talking when they get into the cab, but I love to talk. So when they see me doing autocizes, they want to know what's going on.

After I tell them, we usually have a nice conversation going until I drop them off."

After talking with Hank, I checked around to find out if other people used autocize for similar reasons. And did they ever! My cousin Lorraine David told me she liked autocizing because "I'm unbelievably clumsy. If I start jumping rope, I get my ankles all tangled up. I darn near broke a leg during one rope-jumping attempt. And it's the same for the other calisthenics and what have you that I've tried. Not so with autocize. It's the first exercise program I've come across that gets my muscles in motion without my running the risk of falling flat on my face. You can be the klutziest person in the world and still get some benefits from autocizing."

And Lorraine's roommate, Irene, added her voice. "I've always had trouble falling asleep because I get too tensed up and find myself wide-awake. I hate, though, to take sleeping pills. What I usually do when I'm having trouble falling asleep is get in the car and drive around for a while. That's relaxing for me, but autocize makes it even more so. After an hour or so on the road driving and autocizing, I'm ready for a good night's sleep. I'm sure that autocize helps. I'm getting a double advantage: the exercise and a chance to relax. No sleeping pill could ever provide that."

One of the men I work with informed me that he was on a diet and autocizing helped him stick to the diet. "My problem is eating while I'm driving," he told me. "I always kept a supply of candy bars in the glove compartment. Now when I'm on the road and I get the urge to stop someplace and buy candy, I do a few autocizes. The urge to eat candy, and calories, I don't need passes."

My secretary stopped smoking, and according to her, autocize helped. "Every time I came to a red light or got stuck in traffic, I'd light up a cigarette. It was almost an automatic thing. Half the time I couldn't remember lighting up. Then I made a conscious effort to substitute an autocize for a cigarette. And it worked! Now, when I come a red light, I do an autocize as automatically as I used to light up a cigarette."

As you can see, autocize offers many advantages for every-body. But perhaps the most important advantage is that the program works. My beer gut has long since disappeared, and my wife has lost her double chin. Other people have told me of their newly firmed muscles, and I believe them. I can see the difference. I used to know a lot of flabby, sagging people. Now I know a lot of people with firm, attractive bodies.

What about you? Wouldn't you rather be in good physical shape? I'm sure you would. Well, autocizing can help you, as it has helped so many others.

GETTING READY
FOR
AUTOCIZE

AUTOCIZING DOES NOT REQUIRE SPECIAL EQUIPMENT OR clothing, but it does require preparation. The idea behind autocize is to improve your physical fitness and to make you a safer driver. Because autocize can help you reduce tension or boredom while operating a vehicle, you are more alert and relaxed. Therefore, you are more likely to drive in a safe manner. There is, however, more to safe driving than being alert and relaxed. Good driving habits are also required. Before you even begin your autocize program, learn to handle yourself in a vehicle. In short, drop any sloppy driving habits you may have developed over the years and replace them with good, safe habits.

First of all, sit in your vehicle correctly. Make sure the seat is adjusted properly. It should not be so far back that you have to strain to reach the pedals. On the other hand, the seat should not be so far forward that you have trouble steering. Each time you get into your car, check the position of the seat.

The type of shoe you are wearing may require you to make an adjustment in the seat. For example, if you are wearing platform soles, you may have to move the seat back; if you are wearing sneakers, you may have to move the seat forward. And speaking of footwear, it is dangerous to drive barefooted or in loose-fitting, thong-type sandals.

Once you have the seat adjusted properly, check that you are able to see over the steering wheel and through the rear-view mirror. If you cannot, get yourself a seat cushion to raise your body. These cushions are available in any auto supply store.

Whenever you operate a vehicle, sit up straight, with your back firmly against the seat. Hold your head erect, and place your hands on the steering wheel in the so-called ten o'clock-two o'clock position. Your elbows should be flexed slightly downward. Hold the wheel securely, but not tightly. When you grasp the wheel too tightly, you tense up the muscles in your fingers, hands, and arms. Unnecessary fatigue results. (If you find that you have to hold the wheel tightly to control the car, there is something wrong with the steering mechanism. Have it checked—IMMEDIATELY!)

When you sit behind the wheel in a correct fashion, you

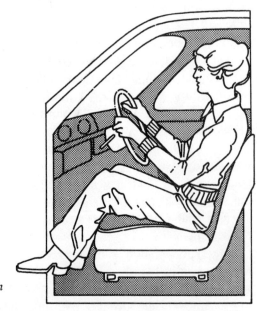

Ideal position for driving

reduce back strain and fatigue. Naturally, slouching in your seat is out. Not only is slouching hard on your body, but it is also dangerous to your driving. Another habit that is dangerous is casual one-handed driving. And it makes no difference whether you have power steering or not. Whenever you are operating a vehicle, keep both hands on the wheel.

Once you are properly settled in your car with the seat comfortably adjusted, fasten that seat belt. Many people avoid using the belts, I know. Usually they rationalize this omission with some silly, and dangerous, excuse like: "Seat belts wrinkle my clothes." (But not as much as you'd be wrinkled if you had an accident.) Or "Seat belts make it hard for me to breathe." (Loosen them a bit.) Or "Every time I release the belts, I break a fingernail." (Open the belts more carefully.)

Actually there is no excuse for not using a seat belt (whether you are a driver or a passenger). Besides the safety factor, seat belts help prevent fatigue by supporting your body in the proper position.

Seat belts are now standard equipment in all vehicles. If you happen to have a pre-seat-belt car, have the belts installed. It's a safe investment if there ever was one.

Another common, and sloppy, habit that many drivers fall into involves the use of the hand (or emergency) brake. Most drivers, particularly automobile drivers, do not use the hand brake. Even when you turn the engine off for a few minutes, *set the hand brake*. And most certainly set the hand brake when you leave the car engine running. Setting the transmission in park or neutral *is not enough*. In fact, the safest thing you can do is never to leave the engine running when you are not in the car. I know a lot of people neglect to set the hand brake with the excuse "I forget to release it." If you get into the habit of setting the brake, you will get into the habit of releasing it.

Speaking of brakes, when you drive a car with an automatic transmission, do you use your left foot for the brake and your right foot for the accelerator? If you do, that's a sloppy driving habit. Operate both the brake and the accelerator with your right foot.

After you have established safe driving habits, practice each autocize given in this book several times. What I would suggest is that you try out each autocize in the privacy of your car while the machine is safely parked in your driveway.

There is, though, one other thing you might want to consider for autocizing—music. While I was researching this book, I was struck by the fact that a good many physical culturists shared one opinion. They suggested that their exercises be done to music. A great suggestion, I think, because music helps one establish a rhythm. If you can work music into your autocize program, terrific. Most cars today come equipped with a radio and/or a tape deck. A tape deck is even better than a radio because you are guaranteed the music you like. Autocizes should be done to what is called mood music, a composition with a slow, soothing beat. When you're autocizing, you aren't supposed to bounce around like a mechanical doll. That's a great way to pull a muscle. Music like rock is just too fast for your purposes. And since the music will be most likely playing while you are operating the car, moving around to an overly fast beat is just plain dangerous.

And while we're on the subject of doing autocizes to music, if you have a portable tape recorder, you can continue playing music when the ignition is turned off. Since I like the idea of always doing autocizes to music without the worry of wearing down the battery, I bring my tape recorder with me. Now, whenever the ignition is off, I just switch on the recorder.

Don't feel, though, that music is essential to your autocize program. It is not. Should you prefer to create your own beat, that's just fine. I realize that many people simply do not enjoy music and that others like to keep their car radios tuned to all-news stations. Autocizing does not mean that you have to give up something you enjoy or introduce something that you do not enjoy into your life.

One final word about getting ready for your autocize program. When muscles have not been used as fully as they might be for a long period of time, they have to be put back into shape gradually. Therefore, you have to plan on working into your autocize program a bit at a time. Right now I can do all these exercises as many times a day as I want to, but when I first started, I could not. I had to take it easy and break myself in. You will, too.

Consider for a moment how many times each you stop, double-park, get in and out of your car, and wait for a passenger. A good number of times. If you were to plunge right in and start doing each set of exercises each time you did something with your car, at the end of the first day you would ache! Believe me, you would.

Therefore, for the first week of autocizing do each set of exercises only once each day. For the second week double the number of times. After two weeks your muscles should be in reasonably good shape, and you can go through the program as often as you want each day. If, however, you feel you need another week or two of warm-up time, go ahead. These are your muscles. Only you can judge how much activity they can take when you have not used them for a longer period of time.

CHAPTER
4

GOING
THE DISTANCE

IT'S ODD HOW A RANDOM STATEMENT CAN SET OFF A WHOLE train of thought. That's how the subject of fatigue began to percolate in my mind. A listless conversation that my boss and I had several months ago turned my attention to fatigue. It was early evening, and we were driving back to our office after spending the entire morning and the greater part of the afternoon with a customer. We had about 100 miles to cover —for the second time that day. During the trip home conversation began to peter out. We both were tired. We discussed the customer and decided he was difficult. Then the computer sales for that year. They were down a bit, but not to the point where we had to worry, especially since a new model would be introduced soon. Then our families were brought up. Our wives and kids were doing just fine. Naturally that old standby the weather was raked over. It was cold and a bit too rainy. You might have gathered we were not having the most memorable conversation in recorded history. My boss, without meaning to, changed all that. Suddenly he introduced an entirely new topic into the conversation.

"You know, Jay," he said, "the other day I was reading in the newspaper about old-time travel. You and I have covered about two hundred miles in one day. According to this article I read, a hundred years ago this trip would have taken nearly a week. Imagine that! A week to do what we've done in a day. Now I call that progress!"

Indeed, that is progress, but I wonder if it's been the best form especially when the very real possibility of fatigue is taken into account. Certainly the time saved is great. No doubt about that. But I was more interested in why that trip took a week. Part of the answer, of course, is speed. A hundred years ago people traveled by horse-drawn stagecoach. Now how fast can a coach travel when it is pulled by six or eight horses? Especially when the combined weight of the passengers is taken into account. Let's say six travelers weigh about 150 pounds each. That's 900 pounds. Then the driver and the fellow riding shotgun. Another 300 pounds. Add to that figure the weight of the luggage. Maybe another 100 pounds. Those poor horses were pulling roughly 1,300 pounds after them. Perhaps more. No wonder they couldn't travel very fast.

But beyond that, there were also the mechanics of traveling. The horses had to be changed quite often. That meant a coach pulled into an inn, and all the passengers went inside while the animals were freed of their burden. Changing horses isn't the fastest operation known to man, what with the unharnessing and reharnessing. More time. But there was one advantage to this mode of travel that we don't have today. The passengers had a chance to get out and stretch their legs. A stagecoach was a cramped way to travel, and a break was necessary, not only for the horses but also for the travelers. In short, everyone on that coach was forced to rest a bit before continuing on the journey.

Today the philosophy of travel is completely different. The whole idea is to hop into a car and drive, and drive, and drive. The internal-combustion engine doesn't need a rest. It can push along at fifty-five miles an hour for hours. And that's exactly how most of us drive. No thought is given to the driver or to the passengers. Traveling by automobile has become something of an endurance test. Just how far can we go without having to stop? Most of us play this little game either consciously or unconsciously when we travel. It's not in the least unusual for people to brag to one another about the number of nonstop miles they covered during a business trip or even a vacation. Vacationers, I'm sorry to say, are prone to drive for ridiculously long periods. This is a great way to ruin what is supposed to be a pleasure. When you drive on your vacation, take it easy. Enjoy yourself. Forget about breaking a mileage record. Limit yourself to no more than seven hours of driving each day. Excluding, of course, time for meals. And give yourself a hour, at least, for each meal. That means if you start a vacation drive at six o'clock in the morning and take an hour for breakfast and lunch, your driving should be over by three o'clock. Even if it takes you a day longer to reach your destination, don't punish yourself by driving for long periods of time.

My brother is a great one for driving hours at a time. He prides himself on how far he can drive without having to stop. He has even rigged up a gadget on his dashboard to hold a sandwich and a cup of coffee. It takes up a lot of room and annoys the daylights out of me when I'm in his car. But, he assures me, it saves time. He doesn't have to stop to eat a meal. Whoopee! My boss is like that, too. He doesn't have the dashboard tray, and I'm not going to tell him about it either.

Getting back to that day he mentioned the differences in travel time, we stopped only once during that entire 200-mile round trip. That was to get gas. Taking a break for a meal, or even a comfort stop, is something my boss hates to consider. When we finally did get back to the office, he told me how stiff he was, how physically tired. He couldn't understand why either. It had been such an easy drive. There was hardly any traffic on the road.

Certainly if he had been doing the autocizes designed for a moving vehicle (the isometric type), he would not have been so stiff and tired. Doing autocizes can greatly reduce the feeling of weariness. But even autocizes done inside the car can relieve that feeling of tiredness just so much. Especially during long trips. Trips of several hundred miles. Trips taken at the end of a hard day. Trips taken at night. Such drives are not meant to be endurance tests, yet many of us try to make them that. Why I'm not really sure; perhaps because it is possible to do it. Yet it is so foolish. No one is waiting at the end of the journey to present a medal for breaking an imaginary record. No one really cares that a trip from New York to Washington was made with only three stops of five minutes each and that they were for gasoline.

To begin with, this physical punishment—and that is exactly what it is—is dangerous not only to the driver but also to his fellow drivers. When a driver becomes tired and stiff, his reflexes slow down. He becomes bored with what he is doing. He pays less attention. Especially when he's driving along expressways. And at night. Certainly a superhighway is a boon to modern transportation. It eliminates the tedious stop and go of ordinary roads. There is no need to worry about intersections. But these wide-open roads with traffic flowing in only one direction can have a mesmerizing effect. The driver becomes hypnotized. And dangerous. It's happened to me. During one long trip home one night I was subjecting myself to an endurance test. I knew I was tired, but rather than take the time to stop and relax a bit, I kept right on going. Traffic was light. Almost perfect driving conditions. But then all those red taillights started to look alike. When the car in front of me flashed on its brake lights, I scarcely noticed until it was almost too late. Those brake lights were just two red circles in front of me. I nearly plowed into his trunk. All that saved me was the sudden realization of what was happening and my power steering, which allowed me to change lanes quickly. It was a sobering experience, and today I am not so cavalier about long trips by car. I stop every hour or so for what I call an outdoor autocize session. Fortunately the modern superhighway is ideal for an autocize break. Rest areas are provided at frequent intervals. So are emergency parking areas. And of course, there is always the shoulder of the road. On the rare occasions when I cannot find a place to stop along the highway, I get off at the first exit ramp and look for a parking lot. Once I'm out of the car, I have a routine which I know you will find useful to combat the mesmerizing effects of distance driving. Here's how it goes:

1. Take a good stretch. Stand as high as you can on your toes, extend your arms straight above your head, and

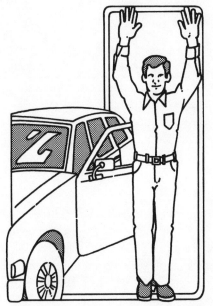

Step 1:
Stretching

inhale deeply. Stretch your body as far as you can. Slowly return to your normal standing posture while exhaling.

2. Inhale deeply two or three times, making sure that you exhale fully.

3. Place your fingertips firmly on your shoulders. Raise your arms slowly so that your elbows are level with your

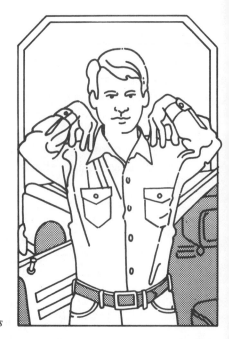

Step 3:
Relaxing shoulders

shoulders. Keeping your fingertips in place, lower your arms. Repeat this action five times.

4. Turn toward the front of your car so that the driver's door is on your right. Grasp the handle of the car door in your right hand. Without bending your knee, kick your left leg back and forth several times. Next, slowly raise your left leg by bending your knee and bringing the heel of your foot toward your buttocks. Hold for a count of three, and slowly bring your leg down. Turn toward the back of the car so that the driver's door is on your left. Grasp the handle of the car door in your left hand, and repeat the same procedure with your right leg.

This whole process takes less than five minutes, and when you are finished, you will feel refreshed and more alert. Five minutes is a small amount of time to invest so that you arrive at your destination in an alert state rather than in physical exhaustion. And when you take into consideration

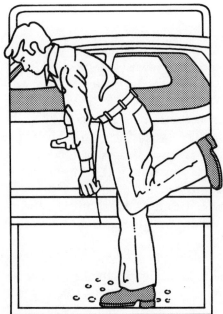

Step 4 (page 42):
The leg stretch

that you will be a safer driver and reduce your chances of an accident caused by fatigue, you will find that five minutes is a very tiny amount of your time.

For your own safety, however, keep in mind that autocizing can only reduce fatigue. It cannot eliminate it. Even though driving while we are overly tired is dangerous, many of us do not recognize excessive fatigue when it comes up on us. In a car there are certain warning signs that appear when we have pushed our bodies too long, that the time for auto-cize is past and the need for sleep is present.

1. The most obvious sign is excessive yawning. Not the occasionally stifled yawn that comes from boredom or the one that comes from being too long in a closed, stuffy area, such as a car with the windows closed. This stuffy condition is aggravated during the cold weather when the heater is running. It is doubly aggravated when the driver or the passengers are smoking. (For more on this subject,

see Chapter 9.) When boredom passes, the yawns stop. And once we leave an enclosed area and get some fresh air, we stop yawning, too. The yawns of fatigue are something else again. They come one right after another.

2. The eyes are also affected by fatigue. They may begin to burn or hurt. Vision becomes blurred. Focusing is difficult, if not impossible. The eyelids have to be forced to stay open. Indeed, they may even drop shut for a second or two. And that second or two is all it takes to fall asleep at the wheel of a car.

3. Fatigue plays havoc with the body's muscle network, hence the drooping eyelids. And the uncooperative neck muscles. When fatigue comes, the neck muscles loosen. The head nods. It is difficult to hold the head up. And when someone cannot hold his head up, he cannot see what is in front of him.

4. An inability to concentrate is another sign of excessive fatigue. For instance, you are not sure where you are in terms of exit or street signs. You are not aware of traffic conditions—is there a car next to you, behind you? Things are just not registering. Along with a lack of concentration comes forgetfulness. You see a red light, but you have to remind yourself what to do about it. And there is the carelessness. You change lanes or make turns without looking or signaling. This is a particularly dangerous state of fatigue because at this point you may have lost the ability to know that you are too tired to be driving.

5. Poor reflexes are also a sign of excessive fatigue. Operating the car becomes laborious. Lifting your foot to the brake pedal or flipping the signal switch becomes a great effort. You just don't feel like exerting the necessary energy. And the truth is, you do not have the energy to exert.

If, while driving, you experience even one of these symptoms, your body is telling you that it is time to stop. When you are in this state, you are risking a great deal if you do not stop for a rest.

As I mentioned earlier, autocize is not meant to eliminate fatigue. Only rest can do that. Autocize is meant to reduce fatigue, eliminate tension and boredom, and keep your muscles in good tone. There are, though, a few things you can keep in mind to make long drives less tiresome—and safer.

1. Keep the windows of your vehicle, both inside and out, clean. If you or your passengers smoke, the inside of the windows and the rearview mirror will become clouded over. During bad weather the outside of the windows also becomes dirty. When the windows are not clean, it is difficult to see, particularly at night, and eyestrain can result.

2. Keep your wiper blades in top condition. If your car has windshield cleaner, keep the container filled with the proper solution.

3. Keep your headlights and your taillights clean. Dirty headlights cut down your visibility. Dirty taillights make it difficult for other drivers to see you or to notice when you apply your brakes.

4. Take the sun into consideration when you start long trips. If you can avoid it, do not begin long easterly drives in the morning or long westerly drives in the afternoon. If you cannot avoid such trips, wear sunglasses and use the sun visor.

5. Take frequent rest breaks!

Now let's talk about these easy-to-do autocizes.

CUSTOMIZE
YOUR
AUTOCIZE

WHEN THE AUTOCIZE CONCEPT FIRST CAME TO ME, I WAS thinking primarily in terms of what could be done inside a car —that steel, aluminum, glass, and chrome box where we spend so much of our time. But however much time we spend in our cars, we don't spend all our time there. This was a point I was overlooking until I got into a discussion with a newly hired salesman. Once Ted joined the firm, he and I worked closely together.

Ted is a very nice young fellow, bright and eager, but for quite a while he was also a guy whom I described as the clumsiest man I had ever met. Whenever we went somewhere together and he drove, Ted would drop his car keys. It never failed. We'd walk toward his car; he'd fish the keys out of his pocket and then drop them. I had to admit that he was very graceful in picking them up. A smooth deep knee bend. To me, though, the most annoying thing about Ted's clumsiness was that he seemed to drop the keys deliberately.

One afternoon we were walking toward his car on our way to lunch. Sure enough, as soon as Ted took the keys from his pocket, they landed on the ground. I snapped out, "Ted, were you born a klutz or did you have to work at it?" I could tell from the way he looked at me that he didn't like my question.

"Whatever gave you the idea that I'm a klutz?" he asked.

"Every blasted time we get into your car, you drop the keys. Now if that isn't the mark of a klutz, I don't know what is."

"Oh, you think so?" he said as he bent down to retrieve the keys. Once we both were settled in the front seat, Ted calmly asked me, "How many times each day do you think I get into my car?" I had no idea, and I told him so. Personally, I wasn't all that interested either. "I kept track once," Ted explained. "For a whole week. It averages out to twelve times a day. Twelve times every single day I get into my car. That's a lot of times." I couldn't see where this conversation was leading and told him so.

"Jay, would it surprise you if I told you that I drop those keys deliberately?"

"No, it wouldn't. In fact, I've suspected you of doing just that. What's the idea behind it?"

"Because when I drop the keys, I have to pick them up. It's a form of exercise. I do about twelve deep knee bends every day. Twelve deep knee bends I wouldn't otherwise get around to doing."

Now that Ted had explained what he was doing, I couldn't consider him a prize klutz anymore. Just the opposite. It was a darn good idea. One that would fit in very well with my autocize scheme. Getting into a car had never struck me as having the possibility for an exercise. Now it did. More time to be put to very good use. There was just one drawback that I could see. "Do many people call you clumsy?" I wanted to know.

"To tell you the truth, you're the first one who's ever made a crack about it. Most people really don't watch others. Somebody drops his car keys. So what? And if I were asked, I'd explain as I just did. I'm more concerned about doing the deep knee bend properly than about what others think anyway."

Ted made a good point there. No form of exercise is going

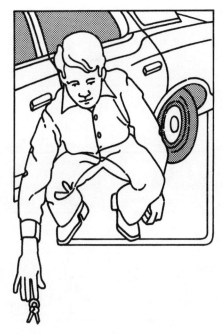

*Pick up keys with
a deep knee bend*

to get you very far if it isn't done right. Here's how to do a deep knee bend: Pull your stomach muscles in gently but firmly. Leave your arms loose at your sides. Keeping your back and shoulders straight, bend slowly from your knees. Pick up the keys and slowly rise. As you go down, inhale. As you stand up, exhale.

There are a few safety measures to bear in mind: If your car is parked on the street, always remember to do this exercise on the passenger's side of the car. There is no reason to do exercises to keep fit if you are going to run the risk of being sideswiped by an oncoming car.

Dropping the car keys each time you want to get into the automobile got me to thinking that there must be other ways of making maximum use of the car for exercise. I thought about it one evening, and it occurred to me that a car comes equipped with a trunk. That trunk can be a wonderful exercise gadget. Before getting into your car, open the trunk. Then stand on your toes, as high as you can go. Spread your

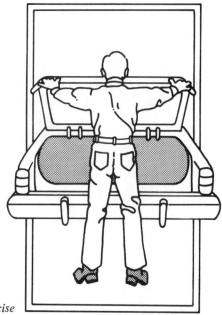

The trunk exercise

arms out so each hand is reaching toward one side of the trunk. Now slam it down as hard as you can. This is another exercise that you can do without people wondering what you are doing. After all, what's so odd about someone slamming down a trunk? People do it all the time. You can also, if you like, do the same thing with the hood of your car.

This idea of exercising while outside the car eventually led to what I've come to call the Supermarket Shuffle. This particular autocize came to me one Saturday morning when my son and I did the grocery shopping for my wife. Kim had plans of her own, and no way could she fit in the weekly trip to the supermarket. Craig and I finally finished up with eight bags of groceries stacked into two shopping carts. Once we were outside the store, my son cheerfully announced that he had to run over to the stationery store and pick up a few things. I decided to wait for him. Having nothing better to do while Craig ran his errand, I started watching the people who were coming and going. One woman came out of the store pushing a cart full of groceries, two or three bags. With considerable skill, she maneuvered the cart down the ramp and across the parking lot to her car, where she loaded the groceries into it. Like a lot of other people, she pushed the cart to one side, hopped into her car, and drove off.

Another man came out of the store. He went one better. He didn't even bother to push the cart across the parking lot. He left the groceries in front of the store and strolled over to his car. Then he drove back to where he had left the cart and loaded his groceries into the vehicle. The minimum mount of physical effort. No doubt about that. He may even have saved a few minutes of time.

That's what got me to thinking about the Supermarket Shuffle. It struck me as being a terrific opportunity for more exercise. Why not carry those bags of groceries over to the car instead of wheeling them or bringing the car over to the grocery cart? A lot of extra benefits could be derived from toting bags of groceries, and it would only take a few extra minutes if the whole thing were handled carefully.

I say carefully because the first time I mentioned carrying bags of groceries over to the car, a friend of Kim's nearly passed out. "I usually have at least seven bags of groceries," she said with a gasp. "You expect me to carry that kind of load? And then you have the nerve to tell me that it will only take a few extra minutes. What about bad weather? The bags would be soaked through if I carried them across the parking lot in the rain. Come off it!"

These are perfectly valid complaints. I admit that. But I said this could be a valuable form of exercise if it were handled properly. A certain amount of common sense is required. That's all. There's no reason to tote bags of groceries around in the rain. But does it rain every single time you go for your groceries? On those days when the weather is absolutely impossible, do whatever is easiest for you. But be honest with yourself, too. Are you not carrying those groceries because it is pouring rain or only because it looks as if it might rain?

As for having a lot of grocery bags, who said that you had to carry them all to your car? Why not carry two or three bags and wheel the rest? And check to see if you have a lot of bags because you are underloading the bags. Those of you who do your own packing at the supermarket may be putting a few bars of soap, a can of peas, and a roll of paper towels in one bag. Make sure the bags are filled up. But don't go to the opposite extreme and overload each bag. This is meant to be an exercise, not an endurance test.

Now for the actual carrying. For the heavier bags, take one at a time. Pull your stomach muscles in, but not too tightly. Hold the bag firmly in your arms, and walk at a comfortable pace. For the lighter bundles, carry two at a time. Make sure the bags are approximately the same weight. Cradle the bags in your arms. Now you're all set.

You can also get yourself into shape while keeping your car safe. As you probably know, your car comes equipped with four shock absorbers. Most drivers assume the shocks are there to give a smooth ride on a bumpy road. They do more than that. They *are* essential if you are to maintain control of your vehicle; shock absorbers keep the wheels on the ground. When the shocks are in poor condition, a vehicle will:

1. Lean heavily while taking corners;
2. "Nose-dive" while stopping;
3. Have steering vibrations;
4. Be difficult, if not impossible, to control while in motion.

It's a good idea to check your shock absorbers once a month. And while you're at it, you can autocize.

Place your hands, one over the other, palms down, on the

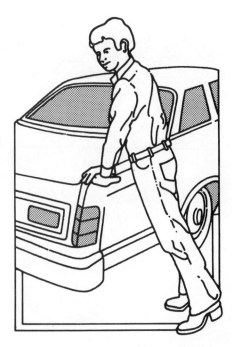

*Checking
shock absorbers*

fender. Pull your stomach in, gently but firmly. Stand on your toes, and use your hands to push down on the fender. Stop. Do this for each fender—but give only one good push. If the shocks are good, the suspension will return quickly. When the shocks are worn, the car will bounce several times before stopping. Worn shocks should be replaced at once.

And while we're discussing shocks, which have to do with the wheels, let's talk about every driver's nightmare—a flat tire. I guess every driver is going to have to change at least one tire, and he might as well get some physical benefit out of it.

Before you start, take the lug wrench. Grasp it firmly with both hands. Extend your arms straight out in front of you. Pull your stomach in, and stand on your toes. Inhale deeply. Hold this position for a count of five. Lower yourself as you exhale. This autocize not only firms the muscles of your arms, legs, and abdomen but also releases the anger you will probably feel when you find you have a flat.

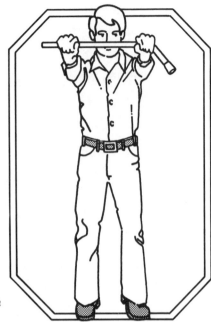

Grasp lug wrench firmly (page 55)

Pull your stomach in while you remove the hubcap and loosen the lug nuts. You can also tense the muscles in your arms as you first loosen and later tighten the lug nuts. The important thing, though, is to keep your abdominal muscles in during the entire tire-changing process.

These outside autocizes provide a nice break in your exercise routine and make for the maximum use of your car. As long as modern civilization has made us so dependent on the automobile, we might as well get the most out of the vehicle. Getting the most also depends on what type of car you drive and how you drive it. I doubt that you will be able to do every single autocize in this book every single day. You will have to select your own autocize program on the basis of the type of car you drive, what you want to accomplish, the amount of time you have available, and the opportunities that present themselves.

The following programs are designed for those of you who are in need of a general overhaul. Autocize is, of course, excellent preventive maintenance and can be applied in a very general way. Or as one of my customers explained to me, "I've had a program of diet and exercise that I've followed for more than ten years now. Autocize is just a bit of extra frosting, because I love to exercise. There's no precise pattern for me. When I have a moment and a leg autocize is what I *think of*, then that's the one I do. If I get a chance to massage my face, I do that. It sounds haphazard, but in the course of a week I find that I do all the autocizes at least once." So if preventive maintenance is your goal, a random selection will keep you in shape. But if you feel you need a planned program. . . .

THE MAJOR OVERHAUL

This program is essentially for men and women who spend at least thirty consecutive minutes in a sedan each day as either driver or passenger. You can follow this program in one of two ways. You can do the autocize program on a four-day cycle. Day 1 is for the head and neck autocizes; Day 2 for the arms; Day 3 for the waist and buttocks; and Day 4 for the legs and feet. Once the cycle is completed, you start all over again. Of course, the cycle is not hard-and-fast. It is tempered by opportunity. Just because it happens to be the day for arm autocizes does not mean that you should miss a chance to do a neck autocize.

Or you can autocize "in order." This program is most useful for those who have memorized all the motions in some sort of personal system of order. My wife, Kim, autocizes this way. On Day 1, when she gets into the car for the first time, she gives herself a scalp massage while waiting for the engine to warm up. She tries to do each autocize for the head and face before moving on to the neck autocizes. Kim goes as far as she can during the day. If she gets as far as her waist (and one unusually busy day, she did) on Day 2, she begins by doing the buttocks autocizes. When she has completed the entire cycle—right down to her feet—she starts the cycle over again.

FINE TUNING FOR SHORT TRIPS

This program is for the driver or passenger who spends fewer than thirty minutes a day in a car, any car. Here I have in mind the commuter who just drives back and forth to a station or the busy mother who is in and out of her car several times a day. You still have plenty of time to autocize if you make the most of your opportunities. Here is a six-step fine-tuning program.

1. Start out by dropping your keys, and use a deep knee bend to pick them up.
2. Get in the car, put the key in the ignition, but don't turn it on. Position yourself properly, and fasten the seat belt. Grasp the steering wheel firmly with both hands. Place your

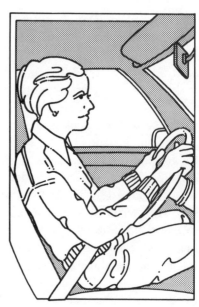

Step 2:
Pushing against the seat

feet flat on the floor. Pull in the muscles of your buttocks and abdomen. Push against the seat as though you were trying to move it back. Hold this position for a count of five. If you are passenger, instead of grasping the steering wheel, place your hands, palms down, on the seat and then push back.

3. Turn the ignition on. While the engine warms up, give yourself either a facial or a scalp massage.

4. Smile broadly as you drive to the station.

5. If you do not have a stop sign or a red light on your way to the station (how lucky can you get!), imagine one after you pull into your parking space. Turn your head to

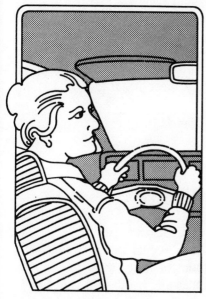

Step 5:
Turning head from
left to right

your left as far as it will go, and hold for a count of five. Then turn your head to your right, again for a count of five. This is a good way not only to firm your neck but also to check that your car is positioned correctly.

6. Turn off the ignition, but before you leave the car, rotate your ankles five times.

Repeat this process when you get into your car in the evening with one change. If you have done the scalp massage in the morning, do the face massage in the evening. For those of you who are in and out of your car each day, repeat this program at least twice. Of course, you can do it as many times as you wish, but to be effective, it should be done a minimum of two times.

AUTOCIZES FOR FUEL ECONOMY AND GLAMOUR

Many people, I realize, drive little cars. Some do so because they prefer the fuel economy of compacts and the fact that these cars are easy to maneuver. Others prefer low-slung sports models because of their glamour. However good on gas or glamorous compacts and sports models are, they are tight on space. While most of the autocizes in this book can be done in any model vehicle, these autocizes are designed to be done when your space is restricted and you are not actually operating the vehicle.

1. With your legs against the seat, place your feet together and flat on the floor. Raise them up on your toes. Push your toes against the floor. Hold for a count of five, and lower your feet. This is good for leg muscles as well as your feet.

2. With your hands resting at the bend of your elbow, swing your arms gently back and forth ten times.

3. Place your fingertips on your shoulders, and bring your elbows together. Hold for a count of five.

4. Lace your fingertips together and try to pull your hands apart. Resist for a count of five. (Remove your rings, if you wear any, before doing this autocize.)

TRAINS AND PLANES

Although it often seems that way, the automobile is not our only means of transportation. There are trains and planes

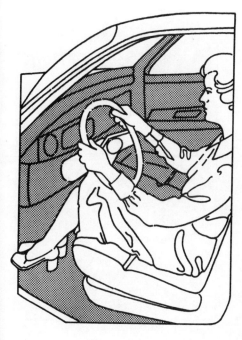

*Step 1 (page 60):
Pushing toes
against the floor*

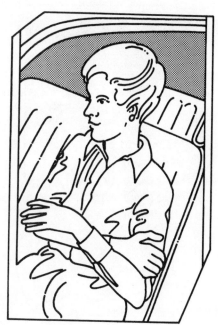

*Step 2 (page 60):
Swinging the arms*

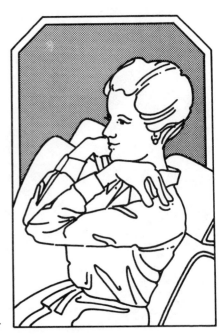

Step 3 (page 60):
Bringing elbows together

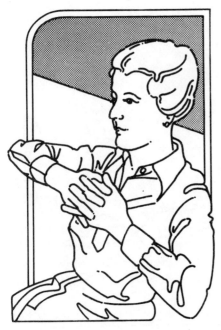

Step 4 (page 60):
Lacing fingers together

to consider. Any autocize meant to be done while the vehicle is not in motion can be done while you are using another form of transportation. The head and face autocizes can present a problem if you're shy and would prefer not to attract attention. Several people, though, have assured me that it is a great way to start a conversation with your seat parner and relieve the tedium of a long trip. For those of you who are not interested in conversation, there is always the washroom for the facial autocizes.

There are also a few more autocize types of motion that are more suited to a train or plane than a car.

1. Marching—Start out with your feet flat on the floor. Raise one foot about four inches; hold, and lower it. Then raise the other, and lower it. Keep this up as long as you like. This is good for the thighs.

2. Jumping—This is a variation on marching and is also good for the thighs. Again, place your feet flat on the floor. Raise them, together, about four inches off the floor. Lower them. Do this as often as you like.

3. Pull your stomach in. Bend down from your waist until your fingers touch the toes of your shoes. Do this three times. (This is not meant to be done after you have eaten a full meal or if you are susceptible to motion sickness.)

4. Get up and walk around whenever you can.

5. Make a point of storing things on the overhead racks. Stretch while placing and retrieving the articles.

6. When you have a reclining seat, push it back as far as it will go. Stretch your legs out. Brace your hands against the armrests. Raise yourself about two inches off your seat. Do this twice. It's great for your arms.

One last program note: Your own personal goals are important, too. Fortunately no two people ever have exactly the same build or figure concerns. Some of you may be displeased with the condition of your legs, but perfectly satisfied with the rest of your body. Therefore, if there are certain areas of your figure that are not up to snuff, you can concentrate on doing the autocizes for this area.

All you have to do is work out your own autocize program. Arrange to customize your autocize. If you find that you want and are able to do all the autocizes in the course of a day or over several days, wonderful. If you find that you do not have the opportunity to do some autocizes daily, not to worry. A chance will come your way. When the opportunity for an autocize appears, take it. The chance, fortunately, to do *some* autocizes will turn up every day. For instance, every driver is bound to hit at least one red light and one stop sign in the course of a day. Therefore, the opportunity for the chin and neck autocizes will appear daily.

Your personal needs and goals, however, are most important. Like any sound, long-lasting exercise program, autocize is for your benefit; you are not for the benefit of autocize!

CHAPTER
6

THE MARVEL
OF
MUSCLES

SINCE THE PRIMARY PURPOSE OF AUTOCIZE IS TO TIGHTEN flabby muscles, we would do well to know something about these muscles we have. Most of us know very little, if anything, about the body's network of muscles. Many of us are not even aware of how much we depend on them. We humans do not make a move or a gesture or perform any activity that does not require at least one pair of muscles working together.

These things we call muscles are found only in animal life, and we humans have about 639 of them. Taken all together, muscle tissue constitutes about 45 percent of the body. Think of that! Nearly half of every human being is made up of muscle tissue. No wonder weak and flabby muscles are noticeable. This vital network is divided into two categories— the voluntary and the involuntary. Or at least those are the more common designations. The fancier terms are striped and unstriped muscles. These terms came about because of the way the muscle tissue looks.

Striped, or voluntary, muscles, as I prefer to call them, are so named because they have a structural makeup that seems to be a series of stripes. Conversely, unstriped, or involuntary, muscles, lack the striped appearance characteristic of voluntary muscle tissue. Because striped muscles are found only in the higher forms of animal life and also have a more complicated cellular structure than unstriped muscles, scientists believe that our voluntary muscles are a fairly recent development on the evolutionary chain.

Voluntary muscles are exactly what the term implies. They produce movement over which we have complete control. We decide when and where we will activate these muscles. Standing up and sitting down are perfect examples. Think about that for a moment. Chances are that in order to read this book, you are sitting down. As long as you are free of any muscular disease, you will not stand up until you consciously decide to rise.

Of course, sitting and standing are not the only voluntary movements we engage in. Walking, running, lifting, reaching, pulling—all are voluntary movements. Any activity you can stop or start at will is voluntary. Driving, too, requires the use of voluntary muscles. Every time you turn the wheel, depress the accelerator or brake, or perform any road maneuver, your voluntary muscles do the work. When you autocize, you will be using your voluntary muscles.

Involuntary muscles cannot be exercised as such because we have no control over them. The action of the heart is a perfect example of an involuntary muscle in action. Usually, though, when I describe the heart as an involuntary muscle, this statement is challenged, and not because the heart is "different." The heart is a crossbreed muscle. It is an involuntary muscle, but it is also composed of striped tissue, as are the voluntary muscles. When I am challenged on whether or not the heart is an involuntary muscle, I usually hear something like: "But I can hold my breath and make my heart stop." Yes, it is true that you can hold your breath and *slow* down the supply of oxygen to your heart; this, in turn, will *slow* down the beat. You can also speed up the beat through rigorous exercise. If the oxygen supply is decreased, however, what happens? You faint; that is what happens. Once you pass out, that involuntary muscle starts up again. It only seems as though you controlled your heart-beat. In the end, the heart functions without our control.

Indeed, all our vital functions are controlled by involuntary muscles. One such function is digestion. When we eat any food, only the first three steps are under our direct control and require the use of voluntary muscles. The actual placing of food in our mouths, the chewing, and the swallowing are voluntary acts. I guess it is nature's way of letting us know that we can survive without raising a hand; we cannot survive without digesting our food. Once you or I have swallowed something, the involuntary muscles of the throat, stomach, and digestive tract take over.

Voluntary muscles are attached to bone tissue and work by contracting and expanding, but in only one direction. As we reach out for something, the necessary muscles expand forward. As we pull in, the same muscles contract backward. These muscles never expand or contract in a sideward direction. The whole process resembles the stretching and snapping of a rubber band.

These muscles are also highly susceptible to stimuli of any sort. Temperature, for example. Walk from a warm room into the cold outdoors of a winter's day, and what happens? We instinctively contract our muscles. We pull them in and tighten them. That's why so many people, on very cold days, walk around with that hunched-over look. Let the opposite happen, go from a cold temperature to a warm one, even one just slightly warmer, and our muscles expand. In short, we relax.

Emotional stimuli get our muscles going, too. When we are happy, in a good mood, we relax, and our muscles expand. But if we are under any sort of emotional stress, the opposite happens. Our muscles contract. They become tight, and we feel it. The famous tension headache that we all are familiar with is the usual result. What has taken place is that we have allowed our muscles, especially those at the back of the neck, to become so tight for so long a period of time that the muscles begin to produce an acid which, after a while, causes irritation.

The whole process of contraction and expansion under stress is fascinating in itself. You've probably heard the statement "I felt as though a weight had been lifted from my shoulders" in reference to the removal of stress. When we are under emotional pressure, we know all too well that our muscles are tight. We can feel the results. The minute the emotional stress is removed, we begin to relax, and we can feel that, too. Each voluntary muscle expands, and the sense of physical discomfiture disappears almost as quickly as it came. Usually we feel a need for sleep. Naturally, because our voluntary muscles are tired. They have been exposed to the brunt of the emotional stress.

These muscles may even ache a bit. A hot bath and a good sleep will solve this problem. Aches also develop when we put underworked muscles to sudden, prolonged use. Any unfamiliar muscular activity is going to cause an ache or two in the beginning. If you are not, for example, in the habit of climbing stairs, the first few times you go up a long flight you will know it. The muscles in your legs will ache.

Some voluntary muscles, though, rarely, if ever, ache. That's because we use them almost constantly. A good example of this are the muscles in our fingers. When was the last time you had muscle fatigue in your fingers? There's a good chance that you never have because there are few human activities that do not require the use of fingers.

Putting your voluntary muscles back in good condition is simply a matter of taking up the slack, as you would take up the slack in a loose fan belt.

Now that you have some background information on your voluntary muscles, why not start to get them into shape. Take autocize for a dry run. Practice the motions where you will be doing them—in your car. Park your car in the driveway, and start fine-tuning you.

THE HEAD
OF
IT ALL

I LIKE TO START AT THE TOP, AND THAT IS WHY YOUR HEAD and face are first on the autocize list. Interestingly enough, very few even think of the head and face in terms of exercise. It's almost as though people believed there are no muscles to be found above the neck. Not so. If it were not for facial muscles, we could not smile, laugh, wink, or blink. We may ignore the head and face while exercising, but otherwise, these areas receive a great deal of attention.

All emotionally healthy human beings—including men— have an active interest in personal appearance. Maybe I'm spilling the beans, but a man can spend just as much time fussing in front of a mirror as a woman can. Especially today when beards and mustaches are so much in vogue. And men have also been known to cringe at the sight of crow's-feet and forehead furrows, all those little telltale lines that remind us that we are no longer teenagers.

Not that anyone has to have an old face. Those wrinkles and sags are made. They do not automatically appear on the morning of one's thirtieth birthday. And with all the creams and lotions available today, it is a wonder that a wrinkle has a chance. But those wrinkles and sagging jowls keep right on forming.

Good news! They can be avoided if they haven't formed already. And if those telltale signs of age have appeared on your face, they can be stopped, if not partially erased. All it takes is a bit of autocizing.

The normal expression of your face is about one-fourth of the problem. Is it a happy face or one that is sad or angry? It matters a great deal. A face that frequently shows a sad, angry, or worried expression uses muscles that leave those unwanted lines and wrinkles. Not so with a face that frequently wears a happy or smiling expression. There's a little experiment that you can try right now in your car to prove to yourself the truth of all this. All you'll need is a rearview mirror. Make a worried face as if you were in a traffic jam and late for work—an expression that creases your forehead and knits your eyebrows together. By looking in the rearview mirror, you can see very clearly how the damage is done. Wear a worried expression long enough and often enough, and those marks will leave their imprint on your face.

Now make the corners of your mouth turn down as though you were annoyed or unhappy about something. See what your facial muscles are doing? Sort of just hanging there? That unpleasant, unattractive expression can easily become permanent—your mouth will always droop downward.

Now for the last part of the experiment—smile, grin! See the difference? Those facial muscles are being lifted up. The more often they are pulled up, the less likely it is that they will sag as you grow older. Furthermore, the happier your facial expression, the more attractive and appealing the rest of you looks. So remember! Smile as often as possible. But nothing stiff or forced. Just an easy, relaxed smile.

As for those lines across the forehead and the bridge of the nose, quite often they are not caused by worry or an unpleasant disposition. Poor eyesight and the need to squint to see properly can bring them on just as quickly. Should you find that you are squinting because you are trying to focus your eyes while driving, you might consider having your eyes checked. If your sight is not as good as it used to be and is not corrected, those lines will keep right on coming back no matter what autocizes you do for your face.

While we all spend our fair share of time in front of a mirror, we spend more time in our cars. And our faces come along for the ride. Now they can come along for autocize. Especially since these motions can be done while you are operating the car. These are the facial autocizes that I use.

1. This autocize is good for the muscles under your chin. Say the letter *O* several times out loud in an exaggerated manner. Pretend that you are taking speech lessons and the letter must be enunciated clearly and distinctly. Do this as often as you like.

2. Here's another one that is very good for the flesh under the chin and the jawline. Protrude your lower lip slightly, sort of like a goldfish. Now open and close your mouth as often as you like.

3. More help for sagging jowls. Compress your lips together but not too tightly. Move your lower jaw back and forth as many times as you like.

4. Here's another facial autocize to do with your lips together. The purpose is to strengthen the muscles above your mouth. Bring your lips together, and pull them slightly into your mouth. Now push air into your mouth. Your cheeks will puff out, but force the air toward your upper lip. You should look and feel as though you were trying to suppress a burp. Hold the air for a count of three, and release it slowly.

5. More help for a droopy upper lip. Open your mouth as wide as you can, and pull your jaw and your nose down toward your chest. Hold this for a count of three, and do it as often as you like.

6. Smiling, believe it or not, is a great autocize because it strengthens the muscles of your cheeks. There are two

ways to smile: with your lips together and with your lips wide apart, showing your teeth. Either way you do it, it will help your facial muscles. Just make the smile as broad as you can, and hold it for a count of five.

7. While maintaining a high level of alertness, you can also work on your forehead muscles by doing an eyebrow lift. Raise your eyebrows as high as you can, and release them downward slowly. I don't use a count with this autocize, but you can if you wish.

All the above-mentioned exercises, while they are easy to learn, require a little practice. Try them out in the rearview mirror first. After one or two trial sessions you'll have them mastered.

There's a bonus with these exercises for those of you who have occasion to wait in a parked car with a restless child. Do your facial autocizes. Children get a kick out of adults who make "funny faces." I found out that this facial routine can

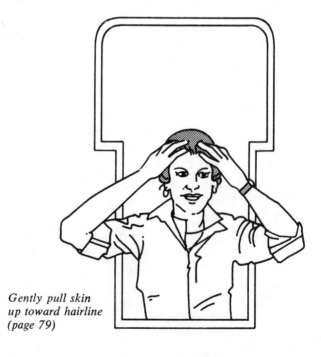

Gently pull skin up toward hairline (page 79)

keep my daughter occupied for nearly half an hour—even longer if she decides to imitate my actions.

Speaking of waiting in a parked automobile, there is another facial autocize you can add to your collection. Spread your fingers open wide, and with the tips gently smooth the skin of your face upward. Start at the jawline, and go to the cheekbones. Having taken care of your lower face, move on to your forehead. Again, with the tips of your fingers, gently pull the skin of your forehead up toward your hairline. Start at the sides of your head and move inward until your fingertips meet, then work backward to the sides. This is so pleasant and refreshing you can treat yourself to this "facial" as often as you like.

By the way, this upward motion should be used whenever you apply anything to your face, be it creams, lotion, makeup, after-shave cologne. Always work from the neck up. Men, when shaving, should also try to work the same way—from

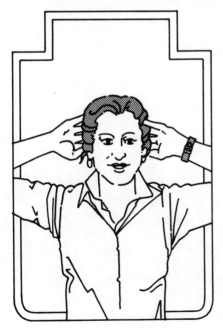

Working fingertips through the hair (page 81)

the neck up. The upward action helps keep the facial muscles firm.

To continue on this subject of waiting in a parked car, if facial exercises and massages do not interest you at the moment, there is always your scalp. It needs exercise, too. Frequent scalp massage increases the flow of blood into this part of your body. The hair follicles are stimulated; this in turn helps your hair grow. Since the massage action causes your scalp to receive more nutrients, you wind up with a healthier head of hair. Although a scalp massage is neither a deterrent to nor a cure for baldness, even those who are losing their hair can still use this technique.

There's a right way to give your scalp a bit of exercise. A lot of people do a massage wrong and therefore accomplish nothing of value. Indeed, they may actually do some harm to their hair. Don't try to massage your scalp by placing your fingertips directly on your hair.

Instead, work the tips of your fingers through your hair

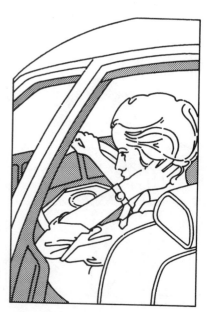

Massaging the back of the head (page 81)

right down to your scalp. Using the tip of your fingers, massage the skin across your skull. Start at the back of your head. Work up and forward past your ears. When you reach your forehead, work back down along the middle of your skull. A gentle, circular motion is most effective and relaxing.

If you often have headaches, especially tension headaches, here is a particularly good autocize to consider. It can be done safely while you are operating your car during tie-ups or whenever traffic is moving at a crawl. Keeping one hand on the steering wheel, gently massage the back of your head, the area just above your neck, in a circular motion.

After a few weeks of doing these autocizes, you should notice a firmer-looking, more smiling you.

THE NECK'S
STOP

UNTIL I STARTED ON MY AUTOCIZE PROGRAM, I LOOKED UPON signs and traffic lights as the curse of every licensed driver in this country. Having to come to a full stop was just one more interruption in the smooth flow of my driving routine. Because these interruptions were annoying, I have to admit that I didn't pay a great deal of attention to them, especially stop signs. I'd sort of stop. That means I never really came to a complete stop. "Slowed down" is a better way to describe it. Then I'd sort of look left and right. That means all I did was glance around. Then I'd zip forward.

Not exactly a safe driving technique. And I did have a few close calls. Autocize has changed all that. Now I look forward to full-stop signs and red lights. Why? What's so special about coming to a complete stop? It gives me a chance to exercise my neck.

A few neck exercises every day can help prevent a couple of common complaints. For one thing, that stiff feeling in the back of the neck that comes after a hard day. Too, that very common bugaboo crepey skin. After I had done these neck exercises for a few weeks, my wife pointed out that I was carrying my head in a more distinguished way. "You look more confident and self-assured than ever," she told me.

That's what comes of having firm neck muscles, and I achieved them by using two very simple exercises. Everyone can have the same look just by remembering that the neck is there. It is, you know, after the face and head the most neglected part of the body.

Who really thinks of the neck as needing regular exercise of any sort? Very few of us, and quite understandably, too. After all, the average neck is working all day—holding up a head. And our heads move all the time. Isn't that right? We're looking around. We're looking over our shoulders. We're looking up. We're looking down. All this is true, but even though the head is moving all the time (or so it seems), we are not really giving those muscles the exercise they need.

You probably doubt this statement. Most of my friends, when I first brought up this subject of neck muscles, took the information with a "Forget my neck, Jay. It gets plenty of exercise." I say chances are very good that your neck doesn't get half the exercise that it needs. And I can prove it. There is a quick test that you can take right now. In your car where you are practicing your autocizes.

Sit up straight. Pull your stomach in gently, square off your shoulders, raise your chin, and stare directly in front of you. Without moving your shoulders, turn your head to your left as though you wanted to look behind you. Now do the same thing by turning toward your right. How far could you turn your head before you began to feel your neck muscles pulling? Probably not very far. While the human head is not designed to make a 360-degree turn or even a 180-degree turn, it should easily make a 90-degree or one-quarter turn. By easily, I mean no excessive pull on the neck muscles. Try it. Are you beginning to change your mind about your neck and the amount of exercise it needs?

Here's another experiment. Stay in your car, and assume the same posture as you did when trying to turn your neck. But instead of turning either left or right, look up at the top of the auto. Again, keep your shoulders straight. Did you feel any muscle pull? I'll bet you did—a lot of it, too. Do you know why? Because those muscles have not exercised enough. Now do you believe that your neck muscles need exercise—just like all the other muscles in your body? Here's what you can do to keep your neck in the best possible condition. First of all, sit in your car correctly whether you are a driver or a passenger. (See p. 29 for the correct procedure.) Sitting properly is a big help. Not only is it safer, but it also aligns your body so there is no undue muscle strain.

There are two autocizes that I use for my neck. They are for two different driving situations. The first one is for a stop sign. It's done like this:

When I come to a stop sign, I stop. Fully. Completely. No cheating. I find that this autocize really cannot be done properly unless I do come to a full stop.

Then I turn my head slowly to my left. Slowly is the key word here. It's no good jerking your head around quickly. That's a great way to pull some muscles. I take a good look at the traffic situation to my left and count to three. I repeat the same procedure by turning toward my right. Again, for a good look at the traffic situation and for a count of three. Of course, it does not matter if you want to look right first and then left.

The other exercise is done at red lights, which I once considered a great time waster in my travels. Now I see them as valuable tools in my autocize program.

Stoplights, as you probably know, are set on a timer for the speed at which the traffic should move. If the speed limit is fifty-five miles per hour, when you travel at this speed, you will not have to stop for any red lights—theoretically, that is. You and I both know otherwise. It is possible to drive along a road and hit every red light. This usually happens when you're in a hurry. And some lights take longer to change than others. This is especially true for a traffic signal that is at the intersection of a primary and a secondary road. As you come along the secondary road and hit the red light, you sit and wait. The idea is to get the traffic moving along the main artery. But you sit and wait on the secondary road convinced that you'll grow old before the light changes. Actually, though, the waiting time is only sixty seconds. One full minute. Not a long period, but you can do a lot in that brief span.

What would you ordinarily do while waiting for a light to change? Stare at the scenery? Change the radio station? Light a cigarette? Wonder when the lousy traffic is going to start moving again? Why not take that valuable time for an autocize? Do an exercise to help your neck muscles.

First, check your sitting posture. As you get more deeply into autocize, you will find that you sit correctly in your car as a matter of course. In the early days of this program you may find that you tend to slip back into the old, sloppy habits of sitting in a car.

Keeping your hands on the steering wheel, slowly bend your head back as far as it will go, and count to five. Bring

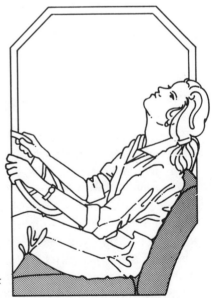

*Bending head back
as far as it will go*

your head slowly back to its normal position. Keep doing this until the light changes and you can go.

Add another autocize to this neck exercise by pulling in your abdominal muscles as far as you can when you bend your head back. Again, hold for a count of five.

As time goes by and you build up your coordination, you can combine these two stoplight exercises. As you are pushing your head back, pull in your abdominal muscles. The count remains at five. The abdominal pull-in can also be combined with the stop-sign neck exercise.

Please remember, though, that safety, while driving, is first. For that reason, the head-back autocize is to be done at a red light and the head-turn autocize while at a stop sign. Do them both at the appropriate places.

While you are toning your neck muscles, you are also engaging in safer driving. Those stop signs mean that you will stop fully and look carefully. While at a red light, you will be keeping your attention on the traffic signal; your mind won't be wandering.

Whether it be a stop sign or a red light, you have to come to a full stop. That means your foot is on the brake. But how does your foot rest on the brake pedal? Lightly or firmly? Most of the drivers that I've been observing let their foot rest lightly on the brake pedal. How do I know that? When a car has an automatic transmission and the driver is not pressing firmly on the brake pedal, the vehicle begins to creep. It moves forward an inch or two. I see a lot of cars creeping forward. When you have to step on the brake pedal, press it down firmly, and then give a tug on the calf muscles. Not too hard. Tighten the muscles firmly, but gently. Do this once each time you apply the brakes to your car.

I'll bet you never thought it was possible to develop a firmer set of muscles while becoming a safer driver.

CHAPTER
9

PLEASING
BREATHING

A YEAR OR SO AGO THE CONVERTIBLE CAR WENT THE WAY of the dodo bird. Instead of being every teenager's dream car, a convertible is now a collector's item. Apparently the growing popularity of air conditioning helped to make the convertible a thing of the past. Now it means that twelve months a year we sit in our cars with the windows tightly closed against the weather, be it hot, cold, or temperate. Driving around in the summertime with the windows tightly sealed against the heat and the air conditioning humming along is a pleasant way to go. We travel in comfort, and I, for one, would not have it any other way.

Now the winter months are something else again. It's cold outside, so we close the windows up tightly and turn on the heater. Maybe even full blast so that the car becomes a nice, warm, cozy place in which to be. Sound familiar? I'm sure it does. But have you ever thought what happens when you sit in your nice, warm car with the windows closed for a long period of time? Quite a bit happens, and not much that is good.

After a while you probably begin to get a bit sleepy. Any extreme of temperature will cause that reaction. If you were to spend too much time in very cold air, you would get sleepy as well. But the drowsy feeling is not entirely due to the warm air inside the car.

You are also in there breathing—inhaling oxygen and exhaling carbon dioxide. Perhaps you have one or two passengers in the car who are doing the same thing. After a while the car is filled with a lot of carbon dioxide, and you're beginning to inhale it. Now to set an even more realistic scene. Let's assume that you are smoking. We will also assume that your passengers are smoking. Again, the air in the car becomes filled with fumes. In short, the air is stale and no longer healthy; this is what you are breathing in. No wonder you're getting sleepy. Your passengers can afford to doze off, but you, as the driver, cannot. And of course, you want every possible opportunity for an autocize. Breathing can afford just such a possibility.

First of all, in the winter always leave the windows, especially the ones in the front, open an eighth of an inch or so, just enough so that there is a constant supply of fresh air coming into the car. The old air can be cleaned out, and the warmth of the heater won't make you too relaxed and drowsy. What little draft does come in won't be that noticeable either to you or to your passengers, and the heater will still maintain a comfortable temperature.

Now for a breathing autocize, one that can be done, of course, at any time of the year. You are going to empty your lungs completely of air. The old, stale air will be forced out and replaced with fresh air. The purpose of this autocize is twofold: to pull in your abdominal muscles and to increase your level of alertness.

Inhale deeply, as far as you can, pulling in your abdominal muscles as you do so. Hold for a count of three. Then exhale fully and completely. Force all the old air out of your lungs. You will know that your lungs are empty when you can no longer exhale. Now inhale again. Deeply. Hold for a count of three. Repeat this process two more times.

Almost immediately you should feel a new sense of alertness. Too, while you are doing this autocize, you are pulling in your abdominal muscles and allowing them to tighten a bit.

This is an autocize that can be done while the car is either in motion or parked. When I am driving with either the air conditioner or the heater running, I make it a point to lower the window on the driver's side every half hour or so and do this autocize. I find it very refreshing. I also find that the brief time that the window is wide open is just enough to increase your level of alertness.

TO ARMS,
TO ARMS

As I got more deeply into my autocize program, I began to talk about it to everyone who would listen. The whole idea of being able to exercise within the confines of an automobile intrigued my friends and neighbors as much as it did me. As I outlined the program, whoever I was talking to would listen intently while I described the exercises for the head, neck, and lungs. As soon as I mentioned the arms and shoulders, I would have my interruption.

"You can't do arm exercises in a car, Jay," I would be told. "There isn't enough room unless you're driving around in a limousine."

Maybe the words would differ, but the sentiments were always the same, and I would always disagree. "It's easy to tone the muscles of your arms in a car. I myself used to believe that a lot of room was required, but a lot can be done in a very small area."

This statement of rebuttal was always greeted with "Okay, prove it." And that's exactly what I would do. These are the autocizes that are excellent for giving your shoulders, arms, wrists, and hands a good workout. There is more than enough room in all cars to do them. Whenever your car is parked, you can autocize your arms.

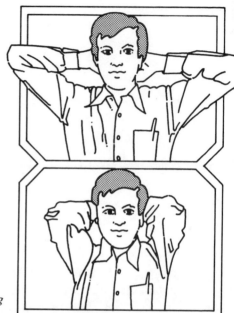

Step 1:
Clasp hands and bring
elbows together

1. Clasp your hands behind your head, and extend your elbows out to your sides. Bring your elbows together slowly. Extend them out to your sides again. Do this five times.

2. Still clasping your hands together, place your hands, palms up, about level with your navel, and then swing your arms back and forth while you count up to twenty-five. All the action of this autocize should be from your shoulders.

3. Touch your fingertips to your shoulders; then extend your arms outward in one of two ways. Extend your arms straight in front of you or to your sides. When I do this autocize, I count up to fifteen. For the odd numbers, my fingertips are on my shoulders, and for the even numbers, my arms are extended outward.

4. This autocize brings the whole arm into play from the shoulders right down to the fingers. It can best be described as climbing an invisible ladder. Reach out with your fingers open, and grasp the "unseen" rung. Use a hand-over-hand motion for a count of ten.

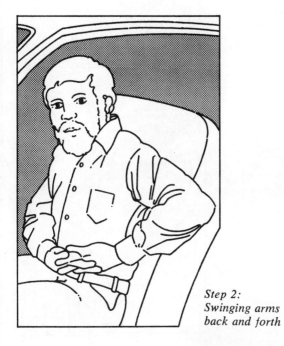

Step 2:
Swinging arms
back and forth

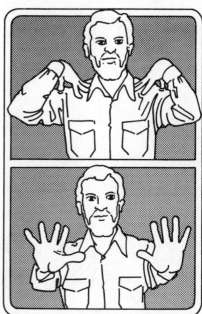

Step 3:
Touching shoulders,
extending arms

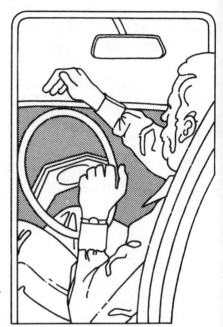

Step 4 (page 101):
Climbing the
invisible ladder

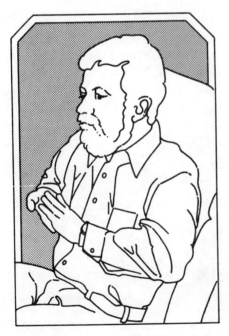

Step 5 (page 104):
Point elbows out
and gently clasp hands

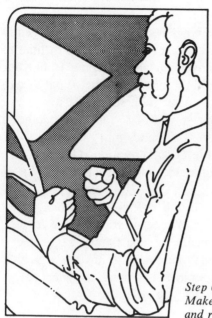

Step 6 (page 104):
Make loose fists
and rotate wrists

5. While keeping your elbows pointed straight out, gently clap your hands. If you have music available, clap in time to the tune. Again, all the movement should come from your shoulders. If you have a child to amuse, a game of pat-a-cake can be substituted for the autocize with similar results.

6. Here's an autocize for your wrists. Place your elbows close to your sides, and form your hands into loose fists. Now rotate your wrists in a gentle circular motion. Go clockwise for a count of five and counterclockwise for another count of five.

7. This last autocize involves a sponge rubber ball. Keep it in your glove compartment. Whenever you think of it, pick it up and give it a good squeeze in each hand.

See, I told you that it wasn't necessary to have a large area to exercise the upper extremities. As long as your car is parked, you have all the room you need.

WASTE NOT
A WAIST

WHEN THE IDEA OF AUTOCIZE FIRST CAME TO ME, I COULDN'T wait to get home and tell Kim about it. Visions of flabbiness fading away danced through my head. All my problems were going to be solved—by sitting in my car! Right after dinner I sat down in the living room and explained my great idea; I even demonstrated many of the autocizes. Kim's reaction was completely positive, and because of this, any doubts I may have had disappeared. That is, her reaction was positive until she asked, "What got you started on this exercise program in the first place?"

"I got flabby. You know that; you were there when Lauren pointed it out to me."

Kim nodded and then said, "Where are you particularly flabby?"

"Mainly around the waist area."

She nodded again. "What kinds of exercises can you do to help your waist when you're in a car? Don't you have to do sit-ups if you want a flat stomach? That's what my high school gym teacher used to tell me."

"There's nothing wrong with doing sit-ups. They do help to make your stomach flat and firm," I said, "but sit-ups aren't the only type of exercise that flattens a flabby stomach.

There are stomach autocizes that can be done in a car. I've given thought to all areas of the body."

"Could you demonstrate?" Kim asked.

However immodest it may sound, I admit that I could indeed demonstrate my stomach autocizes. What I showed my wife that evening, I'll explain here.

1. The first autocize I demonstrated is an old standby, but because it is so important, it cannot be emphasized enough. Pull in those stomach muscles. They should be held in as a matter of course, but when you are in your car, as often as you possibly can, really pull those abdominal muscles in. Then hold them in for a count of five. This is an autocize that can be done even if you are operating the car. The others that I showed Kim can be done by the driver only if the car is not in motion.

2. Give yourself plenty of room for this one by pushing the front seat back as far as it will go and sliding over to the passenger's side of the car. Lace your fingers together behind

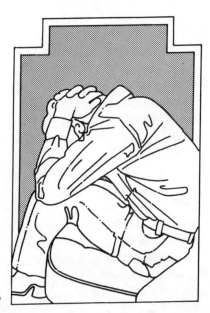

Step 2:
Bending forward

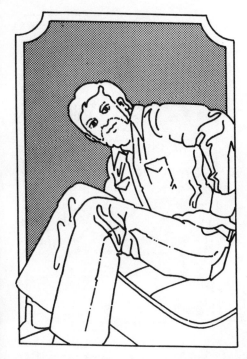

Step 3:
Bending sideways

your neck. Pull in your stomach muscles, and bend forward as far as you can. Do this five times. When you are sitting in the back seat of the car, push the front seat all the way forward to provide the room you need.

3. For this autocize, center yourself either in the front seat or the back seat. Place your hands at your waist, and pull your stomach muscles in. Now bend sideways toward your right until your elbow touches the seat. Return to your original sitting position, and bend sideways toward your left, again until your elbow touches the seat. Bend sideways in each direction five times.

4. Need I mention it again? Pull in your stomach muscles. Again center yourself on either the front or the back seat, and move to the edge. Brace your hands, palms down, on the seat. Now turn, from the waist, to your right and then to your left. Turn in each direction five times. Remember, though, all the motion should come from your waist.

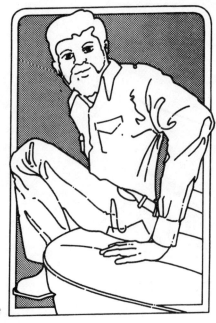

Step 4 (page 109):
Brace hands and
turn from the waist

Doing sit-ups is just fine; I have nothing against them. But there is more than one way to develop a firm, solid abdomen. A good thing, too, because autocizes for the stomach/waist area have more appeal than sit-ups!

12

THE BETTER
BUTTOCKS

IF I WERE TO TAKE A POLL AND ASK PEOPLE WHAT PART OF their body dissatisfies them the most, I can almost guarantee the answer I would receive. Nine out of ten people would reply that their buttocks are the most unsatisfactory part of their bodies. Why? Because sugar settles to the bottom. All that overeating we engage in shows in the tail section. And we also do a lot of sitting, especially with all the driving we do. As a result, many of us fall victim to what is popularly referred to as middle-age spread. Fortunately there is a way to avoid that, as well as the other problem that comes from sitting too long.

I do a lot of long-distance driving; I've already mentioned that. Before I took up autocize, when I traveled to a distant city, I would always try to get home the same evening. To do that, I often had to drive four or five hours without stopping. As long as I had enough gas, didn't need a rest room, and felt alert, I really didn't see any need to stop for a break. Another reason I kept on driving was the road. Sometimes I'd be lucky; there wouldn't be any traffic to speak of. Just clear sailing, and I could glide along at fifty-five miles an hour. Now that was my idea of heaven. I didn't even notice the length of the drive. I'd be home before I knew it.

But once I got home, I would often find myself with what I thought was a unique problem. The first time I noticed it, it was rather embarrassing. Today I can look back on the incident and find it humorous. I had been driving for about two hours, maybe two and a half hours straight, when I finally pulled into my driveway. My wife and two children came out to meet me, and my wife reached over and opened the car door. "I've been waiting supper," she told me happily. "Come in and get washed up. I'll have it on the table in five minutes tops." A chance to wash up and then have a hot meal with my family sounded darn good to me. Despite the temptations of the family hearth, I just sat in the car. "What's the matter?" my wife asked. "I thought you'd be hungry."

"I am," I admitted. "Very. I'll be in the house in a few minutes."

"Are you all right?" she asked anxiously.

I nodded. "I'm just fine. Give me a minute or two to get myself together." I could tell from the expression on her face that Kim wasn't all that reassured, and she wanted some facts, so I gave them to her. "Okay, okay," I said. "If you must know, I need a few minutes because I can't move yet."

"Are you sick or something?" Kim wanted to know.

"No, I'm not sick. There's nothing wrong with me except that my backside is asleep, and I can't move."

The sympathy that Kim had been displaying suddenly disappeared, and she started to laugh. "Your backside is asleep? That's the funniest thing I've heard all week. How in the world . . . ? Oh, that's too much. Maybe you need an alarm clock to wake your seat up when you get home."

I finally was able to haul myself from the car and into the house. All through dinner my wife would look at me and start to giggle. Unfortunately I can't say that I appreciated the humor of the situation. To my mind, it wasn't the least bit funny, but today I can see the joke of it all. Especially since I've learned that other people who drive for several hours without stopping have the same problem.

Any part of the body, including the buttocks, that is subjected to pressure for a long period of time will "fall asleep." The pressure causes the flow of blood to that particular part of the body to slow down. If the pressure is kept up for a very long period of time, real trouble will result. "A few hours" is not long enough to cause serious difficulty.

Generally, this sense of falling asleep affects the arms and legs. We doze off all curled up and rest our heads on our arms. When we wake up, we find that the pressure from our heads has cut off the blood circulation to the arms. Or we sit with a leg tucked under our buttocks. When we try to get up, the same result. The blood supply to the leg has been slowed down by the pressure of the buttocks. Consequently, when we first try to move the affected limb, there is that feeling of pins and needles for a few seconds. Fortunately The feeling passes quickly, and no serious or permanent harm has been done.

The same thing can happen to the buttocks, and for the same reason. Excessive pressure from "sitting" for too long a period, and the blood supply is slowed down. Then you stop the car and find that you can't move for a few minutes. And should you wish to admit, "My backside is asleep," you face a chorus of giggles. It would be better, though, to see that you don't face the problem. It would be even better not only to avoid the problem but also to tighten the muscles of your buttocks. And there is an autocize to help you with both.

The human buttocks is made up of a set of rather broad muscles. You've heard of the famous gluteus maximus, the butt of many a joke? This muscle really exists and is found in your buttocks. Without it, you wouldn't be able to sit down. The gluteus maximus is often one of the first muscles to get flabby. But with autocize you can tighten it up and keep it awake while you drive long distances. You can even do this exercise while you drive short distances or wait for a light to change. It's one of those all-around exercises.

The first thing you have to do is to become familiar with the muscles in your buttocks.

At your first opportunity, perhaps after your next long trip, run your hands across your buttocks and along your upper thighs. These muscles feel loose—maybe even a bit flabby. Now pull in those muscles. These are voluntary muscles, so they will go in when you want them to. You will know when you are contracting these muscles because you will feel it. The buttocks will pull in closer to your body and will feel harder, as will the muscles in your upper thighs. You will also feel a slight pulling sensation in your leg calves. Don't try to walk while you have these muscles contracted. It will be a stiff gait because you won't be able to flex your knees. Now sit down in a relaxed position. Contract your buttocks muscles. You will be able to feel them move inward.

This flexing of the gluteus maximus is an autocize you can do while driving. It can be done in one of two ways. Either you can keep the flexing up in a continuous rhythm (to the beat of any music you happen to be listening to) or you can flex the muscles and hold them in for a count of five. This exercise does not interfere in any way with your driving, so you can do it whenever you feel like it. The more often you do it, the better because the contraction and expansion of the gluteous maximus keep the blood circulating through the buttocks so they won't "fall asleep."

Two things to keep in mind, though. This particular autocize is best done with the abdominal muscles expanded. Relax your stomach. And while sitting, you will not feel your thigh or calf muscles contracting. You will, however, derive the benefits of this autocize, and that's the whole idea.

THE LEGS
AT LAST

"*Yecch!* Do you realize that summer's almost here again? I hate the warm weather," a young feminine voice announced. An interesting remark, and I pricked up my ears to hear more.

Another voice, equally young and feminine, asked, "Why? What's wrong with summer? It's my favorite time of year. There's all the time for the beach. No more baggy, lumpy winter clothes."

The first voice came back with: "The clothes! That's exactly what I don't like about summer. All those skimpy things like bathing suits, shorts, little nothing dresses."

"What have the clothes got to do with it?" the second voice asked. I was curious about that myself.

"Summer clothes show off my fat legs!" the first voice explained. "I've got awful-looking legs and ankles. At least during the cold weather I can hide them under pants and boots."

Ordinarily I don't eavesdrop, but the day I overheard this conversation I was in a diner having my lunch and was alone. The two young women who were talking were in the next booth where I couldn't help overhearing them. Besides, it was an interesting conversation. I picked up some ideas for autocizes. It reminded me how important legs, ankles, and feet are. Especially to women.

The dictates of fashion have made attractive legs, ankles, and feet almost essential. Gone, and we hope forever, are the days when the female form was hidden away in floor-length skirts, thick stockings, and high-button shoes no matter what the weather. Now there is a wide choice of easy-to-wear, casual clothing.

Yet something can be said for those bulky, matronly outfits of yesterday. They did, at least, cover figure flaws like unattractive legs. Today's styles don't permit that. And while women do worry about their legs, that doesn't mean that the masculine leg is free of faults. Nor does it mean that men don't worry about their legs.

Over the years the amount of exercise our legs receive has fallen off considerably. Modern living has seen to that. Walking is no longer the way to go, and why should it be when we have cars? But there was a time when a car offered its share of action for the "lower extremities." That was back in the days when most cars came with standard transmissions. It was necessary to let a clutch in and out. Two feet were needed to operate an automobile, and with the driving conditions back in those days, both feet got their share of exercise.

Not so today. Only one foot is really necessary—thanks to automatic transmission. And even that one foot doesn't have to work very hard. With a light touch on the accelerator, the car goes from zero to fifty in a few seconds. A gentle push on the power brake brings the car to a smooth stop. In fact, it had better be a gentle push, or you and a passenger will go through the windshield.

That leaves one leg doing nothing and the other doing very little. Yet it is important that our legs get some exercise, that they be attractive. What can be done about legs, ankles, and feet while you are in a car? Enough that is worthwhile. Most of these exercises, though, are not meant to be done while you are operating the car.

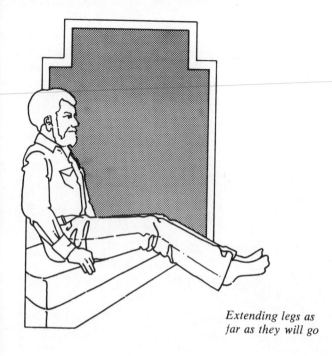

Extending legs as far as they will go

Stretching your legs is perhaps the easiest autocize. Extend your legs as far out in front of you as they will go. Should you be sitting in the front and can do so, push the seat as far back as it will go. Take your shoes off. Brace your feet against the front panel, and then arch your feet and tighten your leg muscles.

To vary this action, rather than stretch your legs out straight in front of you, bring them up to the edge of the seat. Put your feet together. My wife describes this as sitting in "prim schoolgirl fashion," and that's exactly what it is. Now raise your feet up on your toes until you feel your calf muscles tighten. Count to five, and place your feet flat on the floor again. Five times is enough.

You will notice with this latter autocize, however, that only the muscles in your calves are involved. You can actually feel the muscles tighten up, but there is no such feeling in your thighs. That is because these muscles are not involved.

The thigh is usually more in need of firming than any other

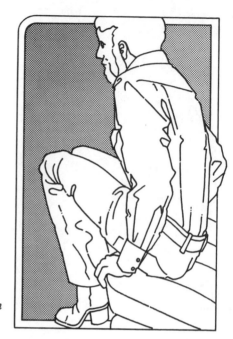

Vary stretching action
shown on page 121

part of the leg. A nice way to get those thighs into shape is by taking a walk. Yes, a walk, but in your car. Lift, in turn, each foot about four inches off the floor, and then lower it. Raise and lower each leg five times. When you first start doing this autocize, take it slowly. Raise and lower your feet slowly as though you were taking a casual stroll. Gradually work yourself up to a fast jog. When you reach the point where you are jogging in place, keep the action up for at least one minute, but no more than three minutes. As your thigh muscles become more flexible, there are two variations on this autocize that you can use.

Place your hands, palms down, on the seat of the car. This will give you the support you need. Bend your leg at the knee, and then raise your leg up until the heel of your foot is on the edge of the seat. Return the leg to its normal position, and bring up the other leg in the same way. Do this five times with each leg. A second variation is to raise

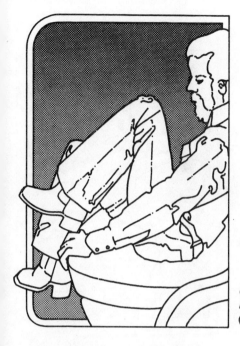

Get thighs into shape by "taking a walk" (page 122)

both legs, in the same way, at the same time. Again, five times.

Another autocize that works on the thigh muscles requires that you be in the back seat. Move over to the far side of the seat. For your left leg, move to your right, and for your right leg, to your left. Raise your leg onto the seat, and straighten it almost to a 90-degree angle with your body. Slowly lower your leg back to the floor of the car. Raise and lower each leg five times.

Ankle exercises are the easiest to do in a car, and this strikes me as ironic because the shape of the ankle has so much to do with the overall impression others receive of your leg. Nothing emphasizes a heavy, chunky leg more than a thin, shapely ankle. By the same token, nothing ruins the line of a shapely leg as quickly as a bloated ankle. But no matter what the shape of your ankle, even if it is perfect, it still needs exercise. Moving only your ankle, rotate each

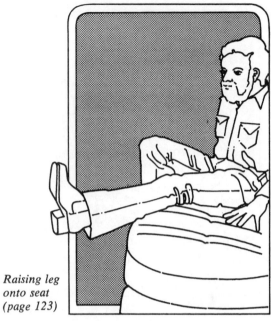

Raising leg onto seat (page 123)

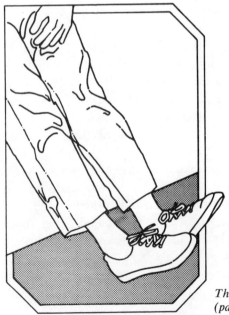

The ankle exercise (page 123)

foot in slow circles. Go clockwise for a count of ten and then counterclockwise for a count of ten.

Once you've taken your ankles for a spin, give them a chance to twist a bit. Place your feet flat on the floor, and put them together. With the heels touching, turn your feet outward as far as they will go, and count to five. Bring your feet slowly back together. As time passes and your leg muscles improve in tone, you will find that you are able to move your feet farther and farther apart. Not only does this action help your ankles, but it also helps the muscles in your calves.

Here is a last autocize that will bring all your leg muscles into play: Place your feet flat on the floor in front of you. Raise your feet up on your toes. Lower your feet to the floor, and then raise them up on your heels. Establish a rhythm while doing this exercise, and keep it up for sixty seconds.

Since I have discussed exercises to tone up the muscles of your thighs, calves, ankles, and feet, that would seem to

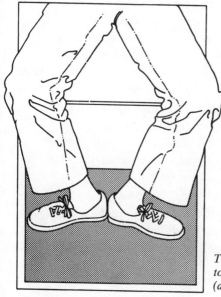

Turning feet outward to twist ankles (above)

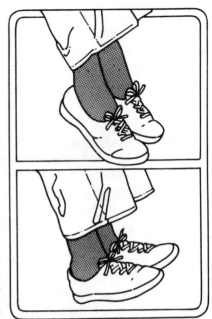

Raise toes,
then heels
(page 125)

cover the legs. Almost, but not quite. There are still the toes. Those ten funny-looking things that don't seem to do much. Toes are important, though, because they help us maintain our balance as we walk, and they need exercise.

My favorite toe exercise is one that has been known to soldiers who stand guard duty. A discreet amount of exercise is necessary if those fellows are to maintain themselves at rigid attention for a long period of time without crumbling. What these fellows do is wiggle their toes regularly.

That is the full extent of this autocize for your toes. Whenever you think of it, give your toes a good wiggle. You can even do this while you are operating the car.

By following this leggy program just once a day, in a few months you will find yourself the proud owner of a very attractive pair of legs. Instead of dreading the summer, you can look forward to the time of skimpy clothes with great anticipation.

CHAPTER
14

STRETCH
IT OUT

When we drive for any length of time without shifting our position, nearly every muscle in our bodies will get stiff. An automobile is the most immobilizing form of mobility that we use. (Any other form of transportation allows us to move around.) Planes, trains, buses, subways all allow us to move around and take the weight and strain off any one particular part of the body. Not so with an automobile. There the driver must sit in place, and the same holds true for the passengers. There's no way they can get up and walk down an aisle to another seat. Stiffness sets in, and with it, tired muscles. Autocize is designed, in part, to reduce this stiffness.

As you drive along, you can move various muscles, one pair at a time. With each stop there is an even greater opportunity to expand and contract your muscles, but every now and again it's a good idea to bring into play as many muscles as you can at the same time. In other words, treat yourself to a good, long stretch without having to get out of the car. To help you get the most benefit from your stretches, I've included my favorite stretch autocizes.

Stretch No. 1. Keeping your feet firmly braced against the panel under the dashboard if you are in the front, or

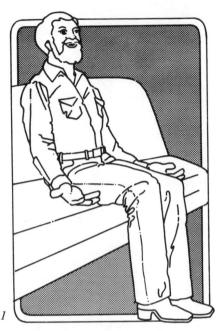

Stretch No. 1

against the floor if you are in the back, lean back in your seat and pull in your abdominal muscles as far as they will go. At the same time put your arms down at your sides. Slowly turn your arms around so that the palms of your hands are facing upward. Push backward with your shoulders. At the same time lift your chin up, smile broadly so that your teeth show, and close your eyelids tightly. Hold this position for a count of five, and slowly return to your regular sitting position.

Stretch No. 2. Again, keeping your feet firmly braced in front of you, pull in your abdominal muscles as far as they will go. Make your hands into loose fists, and bend your arms at the elbow so that your hands are parallel to your shoulders. Using your shoulders, push back against your seat. At the same time lift your chin, and open your mouth and eyes as wide as possible. Kim calls this the Stretch of the Silent Scream, a good name because that is what your expression will be. Hold for a count of five.

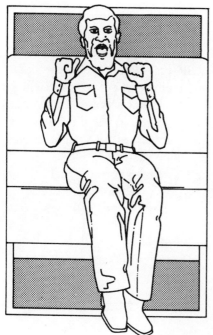

Stretch No. 2

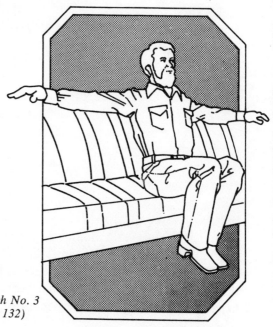

Stretch No. 3
(page 132)

Stretch No. 3. This one is only for the front seat. Position yourself in the middle of the seat. Extend your arms, straight out, along the back of the seat. If your car comes with headrests, then push them down as far as they will go and rest your arms across them. Stretch your arms out as though you were reaching for something. At the same time put your feet together. Keeping your legs as straight as possible, lift them up. Hold for a count of three.

When you do treat yourself to a good stretch, select only one and do it only once. It doesn't take much to relieve any stiffness.

THE FAT
AND LEAN
OF IT

WHEN I FIRST BEGAN TO TELL MY FRIENDS AND RELATIVES about autocizing as a way to firm up flabby muscles, a number of them wanted to know, "If I autocize every day, will I lose weight?" You may be wondering about the same thing yourself. Being "slightly overweight" is almost epidemic in this country. I would guess that the average American is walking around with five, ten, fifteen, or even twenty unnecessary pounds. Most of these "beefy" types know it, too. They worry about it. They are always looking for The Diet but never find it.

But to the question. Autocize is a shape-up program, not a weight-reduction program. It is not meant to bring about a "miracle" weight loss. I cannot guarantee that by using this program, you will shed twenty unwanted pounds in two weeks. Autocize can, however, contribute to a weight loss if it is used properly.

Overweight is the result of eating more calories than you burn off in the course of your daily activities. By overweight, I mean no more than twenty pounds. Anything more, in my opinion, comes under the heading of obesity and probably requires the attention of a physician. Losing weight is a matter of eating less food and using more energy. Every activity we engage in requires us to burn calories. No matter what you do, even while you are reading this book, you are using up calories to provide the energy you need for the activity. The same holds true for autocizing. It requires the use of energy. Obviously some activities require us to use more energy than others do.

Driving a car does not allow us to burn off a large number of calories. And the modern automobile, with all the conveniences like automatic transmission, power steering, and what have you, requires even fewer calories to operate than the automobile of a generation ago. When the amount of time we spend behind the wheel of a car is taken into account, it is no wonder most of us are lugging around "a few extra pounds."

Autocize, like every other physical activity, requires the use of calories. When you do these exercises, you will be using energy—you will be burning calories. Not thousands. Not even hundreds. But some. And every few calories we shed can really add up fast.

Suppose you take up autocizing. Suppose, too, that you do not increase your intake of food—your intake of calories. Then you will lose some weight. Probably a few pounds. But if you were to go on a reducing program and lower your calorie intake while autocizing, then certainly you would lose weight—a goodly amount. If a reducing program does not appeal to you, you can still lose weight because autocize will help you change your eating habits.

The automobile, despite its convenience as transportation, has promoted some very sloppy and calorie-laden eating habits. Snacking while driving is one such habit. More often than I like, I see drivers with one hand on the steering wheel and the other holding a candy bar, a hamburger, or, worse, a can of beer. A whole industry has grown up around the automobile: drive-ins.

Certainly these eateries are convenient and fast. You drive in, give your order through a microphone or to a fast-moving teenager, and then drive off with a meal in a bag. There are just two things wrong with eating like this. The food is loaded with calories, and eating while driving is dangerous. Both hands belong on the wheel when you are operating a vehicle.

Part of autocizing is correct driving posture, and part of correct driving posture is both hands on the steering wheel. Therefore, if you are autocizing, you cannot eat while you are driving. You cannot stuff yourself with calorie-laden foods bought at a drive-in. This is why autocizing can contribute to a weight loss.

Actually you gain a triple benefit here. You reduce your calorie intake while you tone up flabby muscles and become a safer driver. And autocize has still more to offer.

THE MARCH
OF THE
WOODEN SOLDIERS

AUTOCIZING IS MORE THAN JUST ANOTHER SHAPE-UP PRO-gram because it makes us more aware of how we handle our bodies once we leave the car. Proper autocizing, as I mentioned earlier, requires good sitting posture while you are operating a vehicle. When I first started to tell my friends and relatives about the autocize way, a number of them mentioned an "odd" physical feeling when they left their cars. As my sister-in-law described it, "While I'm in the car, I feel all in place. Once I get out, I feel as though my body were falling apart." I heard this complaint expressed in several different ways. Not everyone who was autocizing, however, mentioned this feeling of falling apart. My wife and I certainly didn't notice it. I began to compare the two groups. That's how I discovered what was causing this feeling of falling apart.

The people who complained of this problem were those with terrible posture. While they were in a car, they held their bodies correctly. When they left the car, they reverted to sloppy posture habits. Their bodies were out of alignment, and naturally they felt it. Any misalignment, whether of the human body or of the wheels of an automobile, is noticeable.

No shape-up program, including autocize, will do much good unless the principles become a daily routine. Positioning your body correctly while at the wheel is fine, but if you resume sloppy posture habits when you leave the car, you will notice the misalignment.

People with sloppy postures throw their spines out of whack. They place stress on areas that were not designed to take stress. They forget that they have spinal columns that can take only so much abuse. They hold themselves all wrong.

That backbone of ours that we take so much for granted is extremely important to us and the way we live. Without it, we wouldn't be able to walk around on two feet. The human spinal column is a custom model, and like any custom model, it has to be kept in good shape.

"Wait a minute," you are probably thinking, "what's so special about a human backbone? Other animals have spines and walk around on two legs." Yes, they do, but for only brief periods. Chimpanzees are an example, but even though they appear to be walking on two feet, they usually have an arm dragging on the ground for support. Our natural, normal stance is to be on two feet. Up straight. And that's how the posture problems come into being. We take the instructions either too literally or not literally enough.

A favorite parental injunction to an offspring is: "Will you stand up straight?" Nothing wrong with that on the surface except what the parent sees as straight is not necessarily what nature had in mind. "Stand up straight" tends to mean shoulders back, chest out, stomach in, and head high. Look like a little soldier. Why don't you try this posture yourself? Stand sideways in front of a mirror. Then throw your shoulders back, push your chest out, pull your stomach in, and lift your head up high. What's the first thing you notice about this posture? It's uncomfortable, isn't it? Try moving your arms. They don't work as well as they should. The movements are jerky and stiff.

Now take a look at something else: that curve in your spine. It's pronounced and unattractive. The truth is, you weren't meant to stand like this. And not even soldiers stand this way. Their backs are straight; they don't have unsightly curves.

As for slouching, a common posture problem, that can

also be uncomfortable, again because we weren't meant to stand that way. Nature designed the model, the human body, to move in a certain way. All we have to do is use it properly.

Good posture, standing properly, is not hard at all. It is just a matter of getting all of you into proper alignment. Your body weight is meant to be distributed evenly between both your legs. Throwing your weight entirely on one leg not only puts a strain on that leg but also puts your spine at an angle.

Once the weight has been evenly distributed, then tuck in your buttocks. By doing this, you will push your pelvic bones slightly forward, where they belong anyway. You will also have a backside that seems smaller than it is. Too, this buttocks pull-in helps tighten the muscles in this area.

The abdominal muscles get pulled in next. Again, by pulling in your stomach, you are tightening flabby muscles. Moving up the torso, we come to the shoulders. They are meant to be centered over the pelvic bones, not thrown back so that the blades are almost touching each other. The head

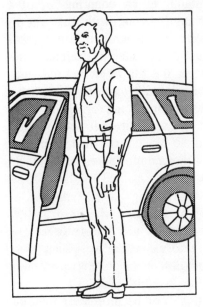

Standing properly

and neck should balance comfortably on the backbone, neither too far forward nor too far back. Keeping your head and neck in proper position prevents a double chin, and it also keeps the neck muscles in good shape.

Now for walking, an activity which a lot of people do wrong. I see so many people walking with their knees stiff and their toes pointing outward. They are also putting all their weight on the heels of their feet.

The stiff-kneed walk is all wrong. You are not a wooden soldier or a wind-up doll. To walk properly, your knees should be slightly flexed. Your toes shold be pointed straight ahead. With each step, your weight should rest on the balls of your feet.

The same guidelines apply to going up and down stairs. Put one foot, the whole foot, on the stair. Bend your knees ever so slightly as you mount the stairs. The upper part of your body should be aligned with your hips.

The best way to develop a good posture for good muscle tone, in my opinion, is that old finishing-school exercise walking around with a book balanced on your head. Not a heavy book, of course. Something light. A paperback will do nicely. Frankly, I prefer a soft-covered book. Should it fall off your head, it won't do much harm. Get yourself into the right posture, place the book on the top of your head, and walk across the room. If the book stays on your head, your posture is correct. If it does not, go back and try again. Keep using the book exercise until good posture becomes second nature to you. And when it does, don't be surprised if your vague backaches fade away. Many backaches have their origins in sloppy posture.

Bending, lifting, pushing, and pulling have a ritual, too. The most common error most of us make when engaged in these movements is to keep our knees stiff. Those knees are flexible—and this is important to remember whenever it is necessary to bend, lift, pull, or push. Bend your knees.

While practicing your posture exercise, let's assume that the book fell off your head (and not because your posture was bad—you were startled by a noise and moved too quickly). How would you go about retrieving that book? Would you bend down from your waist without flexing your knees? Or would you lower yourself by bending your knees completely, sort of in deep knee bend fashion? If you answered with the first choice, you are not alone, but you are not right either. Most people, though, would do exactly that, and all the stress is placed on the back. When you bend at the knees, the leg and thigh muscles share the work. Those muscles also get some exercise.

Anytime you have to bend, whether it is to pick something up, plug in an appliance, or put something away, bend from your knees. By the way, tying your shoes by bending over at the waist is not the way to do it. Sit down, and bring your foot up to you.

There's even a proper way to sleep so that your muscles will stay in tiptop shape. A good, firm mattress is the first requirement. A mattress that is too soft or lumpy does not promote good sleep. Rather, it causes the tired feeling that so many people complain of. As for the best sleeping posture —well, this is going to freak out the Freudians. The best way to rest your body and get a good night's sleep is to lie on your side with your knees bent up toward your chest! That's right—the fetal position. When I first mentioned this to my sister-in-law, her mouth dropped open. "I used to sleep that way," she said, "but I forced myself not to. I thought I had a neurotic desire to return to the womb or something, and I didn't want to be considered a couch case!" Well, good news! There is nothing neurotic about wanting to do the best for your body. While the so-called fetal position is the preferred way to sleep, an alternative is to sleep on your back. Flopping down on your stomach for your nightly shut-eye is out, though. Sleeping on your stomach puts too much pressure on your internal organs.

Now when morning comes and you've slept well, it's a good idea to get out of bed properly. Yes, there's a right way for that, too. And it is not springing up suddenly either.

To rise from a prone position, lift your head, neck, and shoulders in one smooth motion. As you are doing this, shift your weight to an elbow. With the elbow as your support, bring yourself up to a sitting position. Once you are in a sitting position, swing your legs over the side of the bed and place your feet flat on the floor. Then stand as though you were getting up from a chair.

These posture tips will help you maintain your muscle tone while you are out of your car. They will also help you while you are riding in a car. There is such a thing as passenger posture.

When sitting in a car as a passenger, avoid crossing your legs. I know this is an almost automatic reflex for many people, but this position can reduce the supply of blood to your thighs by cutting off the circulation. It can also cause your thighs to get lumpy. Besides, it is not the most attractive way to sit. Try to keep your feet resting squarely in front of you. If you like, cross your ankles over each other, lightly. Too, remember to fasten your seat belt. Just because you are not driving does not mean that you can forget about good sitting and safety habits.

The importance of good posture has often been overlooked. When you hold and move your body properly, you are more attractive, but posture is more than looking well. Holding yourself properly for all physical activities makes you look graceful, self-assured—and thinner. People who slump and slouch give the impression of being awkward, dumpy, almost defeated. They are inviting a double chin, dowager's hump, swayback, and a bay window of an abdomen.

Good posture is also the sensation of feeling well. That vague feeling of fatigue disappears. Often chronic aches and pains for which there is no organic reason disappear. And for plain good health, your circulation improves, and because you are holding your body properly, all the internal organs are in the right places. They are not being crushed. So to look and feel your best, stand up straight—like a human being!

CHAPTER

17

THE MOST
FREQUENTLY ASKED
QUESTIONS

No matter what the program is, no matter how simple and easy to learn, and no matter how beneficial, there are always questions. This is as it should be. No one should jump onto any bandwagon without a full investigation of all the angles. The same holds true for autocize. When I first started to tell others about my mobile physical fitness program, they all were interested. They wanted to try it out for themselves. But they also had a few questions. Good questions, too. No doubt you have some questions as well. That is why I decided to include this chapter of the questions I am most frequently asked. Since they are asked so often and by so many different people, there is a good chance that you are asking yourself the same or very similar ones.

1. What if I have a heart condition (or a hernia or weak lungs)?

It depends on what your doctor recommends. Before starting any exercise program, including autocize, you should have a physical checkup to determine the proper regimen for your state of health. Only your doctor can decide what kind of physical condition you are in and whether or not autocize is a good program for you.

2. Can I do autocizes after eating?

Yes, certainly. Provided, of course, that you haven't stuffed yourself to the point of bursting. In that case, the question is academic because you probably won't have the energy for driving a car, much less for autocizes. If, though, you have eaten a normal meal, doing autocizes once you are back in your car will not interfere with your digestion or give you stomach cramps.

3. Will autocizes keep me awake?

They will maintain your level of alertness for a while. Should you reach the point, while driving, where you feel you must have some sleep, pull off the road for a rest. Autocize is not a substitute for sleep. It is not meant to be. When you approach the point of exhaustion, it is foolish and dangerous to continue driving.

4. I know it's dangerous to drive after a bout of heavy drinking. Will doing autocizes help sober me up?

No, definitely not! If you have been engaging in rather heavy drinking, you have no business driving. The autocizes described in this book will not help clear your head, and they are not meant to.

5. Can children do autocizes?

Certainly, if their physical condition allows it. Teaching children to do these exercises often helps restless youngsters to put up with what might otherwise be a boring automobile trip. I find that most children seven and older can be taught these simple exercises. Younger than that, a child may not have developed enough coordination or perception to understand what is wanted. You can always experiment to find out if your child can do these exercises. If the youngster doesn't seem to grasp the exercises, drop the whole thing and wait awhile. But if your child is able to learn autocize, treat it as a game rather than as something very serious. I feel that teaching youngsters to get into the habit of exercise is a good way to install a lifelong and valuable habit of physical fitness.

6. Wouldn't a protein supplement improve the tone of my muscles?

No, a supplement by itself wouldn't do your muscles a bit of good. Exercise tones, firms, and strengths muscle tissue. Besides, if you are following a nutritionally balanced diet, you don't need supplements, protein or otherwise. Where there are any doubts about your diet and its quality, ask your physician. He can tell you if you are getting enough of the basic nutrients.

7. Isn't the best exercise the type that causes you to work up a good sweat?

No, it isn't. And the autocizes suggested in this book are not presented with the idea of making you sweat. This question is often asked of me because it is known that to sweat, the body must use energy. By using energy, therefore, the body is burning off calories—and fat. The reasoning is something like: "Sweat enough and melt pounds away."

A friend of mine took this theory to ridiculous extremes and almost killed himself. Jack was about fifteen pounds overweight. Last summer his doctor gave him a reducing diet to follow, but Jack was in a hurry to shed the extra blubber. Its being summer and hot, he decided to sweat the weight off in a few days. At the first opportunity he got into his car and began to drive around with the windows closed and the air conditioning turned off. The automobile was literally an oven after less than an hour. Jack was sweating all right; he was also roasting. When he finally decided that he couldn't take it anymore, he pulled off the road, got out of the car, and passed out. He wound up in the hospital with heat stroke. Jack, like others who subscribe to this theory of "Sweat off pounds," didn't fully understand the body's cooling system. If he had, maybe he wouldn't have been so foolish.

Sweating is a normal and necessary physical function. It is part of our body's cooling system. But if our sweat glands have to work too hard to produce the moisture, the body has less energy at its disposal for other vital functions, such as pumping blood throughout the system. Furthermore, to produce sweat, the skin must be hot; the heat causes blood to rush to the surface of the skin (that's what causes us to blush and also produces that flush many of us have after strenuous exercise). The muscles are then deprived of the blood they need to function. To replace this lost supply of blood, the heart pumps faster and harder. This extra work load on the heart can, if it lasts long enough, cause a collapse. The sweat glands also run out of energy and stop working. The "coolant" of sweat is no longer provided. We begin to dehydrate. That's what happened to Jack.

No, you don't have to "work up a good sweat" to tone your muscles. Sweating for the sake of sweating is never a good idea. If you have any thoughts about melting fat away, forget about them.

8. Shouldn't women be careful how they tone their muscles?

Everyone should be careful, whether male or female. There is nothing pleasant about a pulled muscle. The women who ask me this question, though, are worried that exercise might cause their muscles to become overly developed. This fear is what kept many women away from a good exercise program for so long. It was actually believed that physical activity was unfeminine. These fears and beliefs are mostly gone—fortunately. With the proper forms of exercise, those designed to strengthen weak muscles and to keep firm ones in tiptop shape, there is no reason to become muscle-bound. The autocizes used in this book are meant to promote healthy muscle tone. I doubt very much that a woman who does them will develop the body of a wrestler, but then neither will a man! Apparently nature wants a woman to keep her soft curves because it is not easy for a woman to become muscle-bound. The female of the species comes equipped with an extra layer of subcutaneous fat. This thicker layer retards the formation of bulging muscles and lets a woman keep her female shape. So one more excuse for not doing any exercise bites the dust.

9. To be really fit, don't you have to lead a Spartan life?

I certainly hope not because the true Spartan life is anything but pleasant. It means none of the luxuries or creature comforts. All the really fun things of life are proscribed. Personally, I prefer to lead what a true Spartan would call a soft life. No, this idea of taking cold showers, eating only vegetables, and sleeping on an army cot with one scratchy blanket in the winter has nothing to do with toning up weak muscles.

I always have and still enjoy a cocktail, a charcoal-broiled steak, a gooey dessert, and an electric blanket in the winter. Exercise, consistent and regular, not physical discomfort, is what promotes good muscle tone. It's too bad that this rumor ever got started because this is what has turned a lot of people off exercise. Nobody in his right mind ever goes out of his way to make himself uncomfortable. And why should he? Creature comfort is one of the things that make life enjoyable. Exercise should make you feel better, not as if you have just come from the torture chamber.

10. How can I do autocizes in the winter when I'm wearing a heavy coat?

Heavy, restrictive clothing makes any exercise, including autocize, difficult. When I'm asked this question, I always suggest that heavy winter clothing not be worn in the car. Now I am not saying that you should run around in a sweater when the temperature is 20° F and the wind-chill factor makes it seem like −10° F. Wear your winter togs when you are out of doors. But think twice about them when you get into the car. You may not need them on at all in view of the temperature in your car.

Even in the summer I recommend that men and women not wear restrictive clothing like jackets in the car anyway. Take them off, and put them to one side. It will also save the jackets from getting wrinkled. When you arrive for a business appointment, you will look fresher if your jacket is wrinkle-free. Who cares if the back of your shirt is crumpled? Your jacket is covering it.

11. Are there any age limitations to autocizing?

None that I know of. This program is for all age-groups, but your doctor should always have the final say. If you have doubts, check with your physician.

12. What if driving conditions are bad?

Dense fog, heavy rain, and blinding snow and icy roads make even the most expert drivers nervous. Therefore, I strongly advise the average driver to stay off the road under such conditions. If driving is absolutely necessary, concentrate your full attention on the road.

These are, as I mentioned earlier, the questions that I am most frequently asked. It is possible, perhaps even probable, that your question has not been covered in this chapter. Rather than be concerned about a particular point, always remember that your physician is the best source of information when you are starting an exercise program.

CHAPTER

18

A CLOSING WORD

THERE ARE CERTAINLY A LOT OF EXERCISES THAT CAN BE done in an automobile (and a few other places, too). That is a point I was most anxious to make when I started writing this book. You also have a lot of time available in a car whether you are a driver or a passenger. That was another important point I wanted to bring out. And now I want to make one last point—my closing word.

Autocizing is, I believe, the easiest way to tune up your shape. There is, however, one vital element needed before you can autocize. It is an element that only you can provide—motivation! To get the benefits of autocizing, you have to make the effort. I can list the autocizes, explain how to do them, and give you hints and suggestions. That is all I can do. I cannot make you do what you don't want to do.

But here's some food for thought. It may help motivate you. Take a good, long look at yourself. Get down to the basics of bare skin, and check out your physique. How does it strike you? Flabby? Out of shape? Chances are you could do with a little firming up, if only in one or two areas. Very few of us can say honestly that we are in A-1 condition. The thighs, buttocks, abdomen, upper arms, and jowls are the places where flab usually takes over. How do these areas appeal to you? Would you like to improve them? Give auto-cize a try. There is no reason why anyone should walk around looking like a human blob of jelly. For one thing it makes you look older than you are. Frankly it amazes me that this should be so when I think of the amount of time, effort, and money people spend trying to look younger. The hair dye, the makeup, the clothes—and none of this really does any good when the bouncing buttocks and the neglected neck give one away.

Autocizing could not only make you look younger, but also make you healthier. That's some motivation! Here's to a firmer, shapelier you!

SUGGESTED READING

Hewitt, James, *Facial Isometrics*. New York: Award Books, 1970.

Kelly, Frederick, *Isometric Drills for Strength and Power in Athletics*. New York: Prentice-Hall, 1967.

Obeck, Victor, *How to Exercise Without Moving a Muscle*. New York: Essandess Special Editions, published by Simon and Schuster, n.d.

Rossman, Isadore, and Obeck, Victor, *Isometrics: The Static Way to Physical Fitness*. New York: Stravon Educational Press, 1966.

Wallis, Earl L., and Logan, Gene A., *Isometric Exercises for Figure Improvement and Body Conditioning*. New York: Prentice-Hall, 1967.

Wittenberg, Henry, *Isometrics*. New York: Award Books, 1975.